Wh **Way**

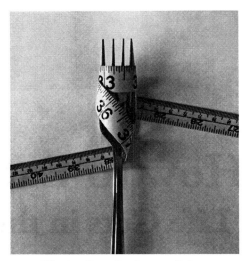

Illustrations By Jeremy Belzer
Cover Design By Steve Sneed & Melissa Zamojcin
Head Shot By Vicki Ochstein

First published by Dog Ear Publishing
4010 W. 86th Street, Ste H
Indianapolis, IN 46268
www.dogearpublishing.net

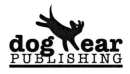

ISBN: 978-145750-237-8

This book is printed on acid-free paper.

Printed in the United States of America

This book is dedicated to the loving memory of my mom, Mirah, who by example, taught me the importance of eating healthy.

GRATITUDE

Food and family go together and without the daily love of my incredible family this book would not have happened. Plus, many of the tips on these pages are from my clients, who have been an ongoing inspiration.

Thanks to Ellen J. Belzer, who would not let me throw in the towel and helped me get this project off the ground. I am eternally grateful to the many rounds of edits by Ellen Taylor, Donna Bliss, Cynthia Grazian, Jodi Shivers, Melissa Zamojcin, Francine Mendelowitz and Miriam Kraemer.

The amazing illustrations were drawn by my nephew, Jeremy Belzer, whose creativity never ceases to amaze me.

Jenny Craig was my first boss and trainer in the weight loss industry. She taught me so much and I credit her for being the best role model and mentor in the world. I respect her for her accomplishments and adore her for her fabulous personality and great sense of humor. Thank you, Jenny, for being so special and for being my friend.

Most of all, I want to thank Mark, my loving husband, for giving me the opportunity to spread my wings and follow my passion. I love you and thank you from the bottom of my heart.

To stay up to date with 'Diet Coach Judy', please check out my website www.dietcoachjudy.com, "like" my "Diet Coach Judy" fan page on Facebook or follow me on twitter @dietcoachjudy.

TABLE OF CONTENTS

INTRODUCTION

How many times have you started a new weight loss program and then stopped because life got in the way? So many things can happen:

- a friend invites you out to dinner
- your exercise buddy cancels on you
- you are invited out for cocktails but you just swore off alcohol
- a birthday is celebrated at work and cake is handed to you

The list goes on and on. You can always find an excuse to abort your healthy eating regimen.

The purpose of my book is to make it easier for you to adhere to any healthy eating program. You will learn how to navigate through the most challenging situations. It is all about having strategies that help you know **WHAT TO DO** and **WHAT TO DO LESS OFTEN.** When you make better choices in your everyday life, the exceptions will not have a big impact on your results. It is important to know that there is no such thing as "bad" food, however, there are foods that are less desirable if you are trying to eat healthy and stay in good physical shape.

Personally, I lost 50 pounds over 30 years ago, and I have maintained my weight ever since then. Trust me, it is not so easy. I could walk by a bakery and gain two pounds by osmosis. I can drink one glass of wine, and the scale goes up the next day. It's so easy for me to gain, I always have to be aware of what I eat or drink.

The strategies in this book have made it easier for me to maintain my weight. I have been gathering these tips for several years while I watched my own weight and helped clients. (Many of my tips come from my clients) My book will make any program easier for you to follow and achieve the results you want. By changing your behaviors, you will ultimately lose weight.

We all live different lifestyles. The challenges someone faces when they travel for work are much different than the challenges of a stay-at-home mom, or a student away at college with erratic hours who is tempted by lots of junk food. There are so many stories and excuses, but the bottom line is: "it is just food". We need food for fuel to keep us going. What we don't need is to eat to excess. In today's world, the advertisers tell us more is better, but our waistlines don't agree. It's time to take control of what you are eating so you can live a healthier, leaner lifestyle.

This is a guide book that gives you strategies on:

WHAT TO DO

and

WHAT TO DO LESS OFTEN

For example, when your friend calls and invites you to an Italian restaurant, you could turn to pages 41-43 and read the tips.

By following just a few of these strategies, you will have a healthier eating experience.

Now, let's get started so you can learn how to eat "when life gets in the way!"

THE ESSENTIALS

In my business, Diet Coach Judy, I work with clients one-on-one to help them reach their weight loss goals by changing their behaviors. In this book, you will also learn how to change your behaviors by implementing new strategies on how to eat when life gets in the way. Before we get started with the strategies, we need to review the basics – the "musts" for healthy eating *every single day.*

Have a plan. Start every day with a good idea of what you will be eating. I know it's not easy to know what you're having for dinner when you first get up in the morning, but at least you can have a good idea if you're eating out or making something at home. This will help you not to exceed your calories for the day by the time you finish lunch.

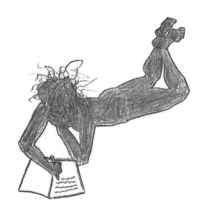

Start a diary. To ensure that you adhere to your plan, it's critical to keep a daily diary. Keep it simple by writing down everything you eat on a small pad of paper, or open an email on your phone or computer and type in everything you eat throughout the day. Save the draft until day's end, and then tally your intake. Or, you can track your daily food intake online. Several websites and software programs enable you to enter what you eat throughout the day and give you the nutritional breakdown of what you consumed. Simply google "food diary online" and you will find several options, many of which are free. The American Journal of Preventive Medicine, Kaiser Permanente Center for Health Research and The National Heart, Lung, and Blood Institute have sponsored studies supporting the importance of keeping a food diary to ensure weight loss happens.

Exercise regularly. Can you lose weight without exercising? Yes, but it will be a very slow process if you don't charge up your metabolism and tone your body as you lose. I encourage my clients to make exercise a regular part of their lives – it's non-negotiable. Whether you work out on a treadmill, use an exercise bike, or walk around the block every morning, you'll get the best results by exercising for at least 30 to 60 minutes, 3 to 4 times a week. This is one essential where more is better!

Keep an activity log and use a pedometer. These are great motivational tools for meeting and exceeding your exercise goals.

Eat s-l-o-w-l-y. One of the best ways to keep from overeating is to eat slowly. Putting your fork down between bites gives your brain time to tell your stomach when you are full, while enabling you to savor the flavor of your food. Taking sips of water between bites also makes it easier to eat more slowly.

Visit the Land of Nod. Getting a good night's sleep will have a major effect on your efforts to lose weight. When we're tired, we are more likely to overeat and make poor food choices. In fact, sometimes when we think we are hungry, we are really tired. This is when we tend to feed our exhaustion, when we would be better off going to bed! When you're tired during the day, take a power nap, a shower, or a brisk walk to wake up. Even stepping outside for some fresh air can help. The more alert you are, the more likely you are to make wise food decisions – and wiser decisions about everything else going on in your life.

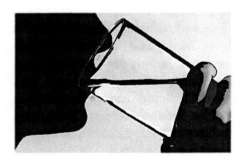

Drink LOTS of water. Among the many reasons that drinking a lot of water contributes to good health and weight loss: it helps you to slow down your eating and, as a result, you feel less hungry.

Don't be intimidated by recommendations that you

need to drink eight 8-ounce glasses of water each day. It's easy to do when you start each meal with a glass of water and drink another glass of water during the meal; that's six glasses right there! For the other two glasses, keep a bottle or glass of water with you at all times. It's easy. You can do this!

Don't skip meals. Whether you eat three regular meals a day or 5 to 6 smaller ones, please don't skip meals. After skipping a meal and waiting several hours before your next meal, the tendency is to overeat. Try to eat before you are starving.

Eating breakfast, lunch, and dinner will keep your metabolism even throughout the day and aid your weight loss or maintenance.

Read this section again and again. These are the basics to living a healthier lifestyle. Whether your goal is to lose weight or maintain your weight, these are the basics that will ensure your success:

> **Have a plan**
> **Start a diary**
> **Exercise regularly**
> **Eat s-l-o-w-l-y**
> **Visit the Land of Nod**
> **Drink LOTS of water**
> **Don't skip meals**

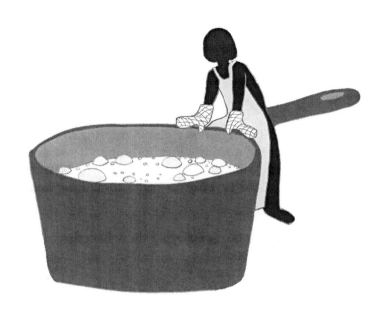

SECTION ONE:

Healthy Eating at Any Restaurant

Can I cook? Sure.
Do I? As rarely as possible!

Working too much, running with kids, making time to see friends, and maintaining your home are a few of the ways "life can get in the way." Lucky for us, we live in a world of convenience foods and great restaurants. Who has time to cook and clean up, let alone shop for food?

For me, it's easier to eat out on a diet. Ordering in from a favorite restaurant is easier than making a meal at home. (If you don't want to eat restaurant foods, stock convenience foods in your freezer for when you are too tired or busy to make something healthy from scratch).

The beauty of eating out is enjoying these benefits:
- You don't have to cook
- You don't have to clean up
- You can order exactly what you want and how you want it served

How cool is that?

And always remember,
Focus on the People and Conversation,
Not the Food!

HEALTHY EATING AT ANY RESTAURANT

Start with a plan. Knowing what you are going to order before you enter the restaurant will keep you from succumbing to on-site temptations. Menus can be found online or you can call ahead to learn about the healthiest options the restaurant has to offer. When you know what to order as you walk into the restaurant, you are less likely to be seduced by the higher-calorie items on the menu or the specials.

Eat your food in calorie order. That is, eat the lowest-calorie foods first (e.g., vegetables), then your grains, and finally your protein. You will have the feeling of being full by the time you eat your entrée; therefore, you will ingest fewer calories. That's why it's always a good idea to eat a green salad before your meal (be sure to control the salad dressing).

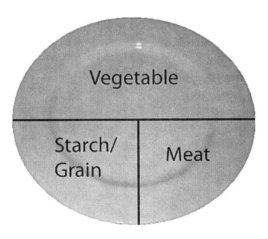

The Plate Method is a simple and versatile method for teaching meal planning. A 9-inch dinner plate serves as a pie chart to show proportions of the plate that should be covered by various food groups. Vegetables should cover 50 percent of the plate for lunch and dinner. The remainder of the plate should be divided between starchy foods, such as bread, grains, or potatoes, and a choice from the meat group. A serving of fruit and milk should accompany the plate.

SURPRISE, SURPRISE!

As a diet coach, I have heard many clients tell me about the fries they *had* to eat because they came with their meal, even though they didn't ask for them. Or the sauce they didn't know about on their fish or the béarnaise sauce smeared all over their filet. The list of "surprises" goes on and on.

The best away to avoid 'surprises' is to be very specific when ordering food in a restaurant.

Remember the scene in the movie, *'When Harry Met Sally'*, when Sally (Meg Ryan's character) is overly specific and takes a very long time to order? It may be annoying, but the results are great – and you are in control of what you're served.

WHAT TO DO:

- **Eat an appetizer as your entrée** – control portion size. (shrimp cocktail is a very low calorie option)

- **Share an entrée** – fight back against up-sized portions.

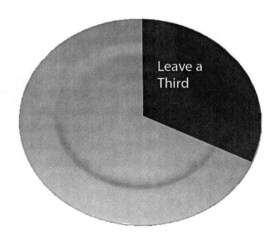

Leave a Third

- **Love leftovers** – you are no longer a member of the Clean Plate Club! Your new goal is to leave a third to a half of what you are served.

- **Drink lots of water** – one glass before and one glass during your meal will curb your appetite and help you to eat more slowly.

- **Record it** – keeping a food journal is a great way to be accountable, and many studies prove it increases weight loss.

- **Know how and how much** – whether you order meat, fish or chicken; baked, broiled, or grilled will add fewer calories than fried or sautéed. When considering a portion size, limit yourself to 3 ounces. Three ounces is roughly equivalent to the size of your palm, or a deck of cards.

WHAT TO DO LESS OFTEN:

- **"Trough" restaurants** – you sat down to a dinner for four, and it is all on your plate! When eating at restaurants that serve oversized portions, immediately draw an imaginary line down your plate to ensure you eat a small amount. Ask for a container immediately so you can eliminate the need for will power while the food is loitering in front of you. If you are not comfortable with that request, then ask the waiter to remove your plate when you have finished eating your designated portion. Take what's leftover home to enjoy for the rest of the week.

- **Healthy endings** – your best bet for dessert is to order berries or fresh fruit. But if a certain cake or pie on the menu is calling your name, order it for the table and have one or two bites. You only taste the first couple of bites, after that, you are building a bicep.

- **Buffets** – assess the options, and then plate your food once. Be mindful of what you choose, and make sure half your plate is vegetables. It is also a good plan to choose only four items. If you take a little sample of several items, the calories add up way too fast.

- **Breads** – have a plan before taking that first piece of bread from the bread basket. Either avoid it like the plague, or enjoy one slice. If your friends don't mind, ask to have the bread basket removed from the table after they have had a chance to take a slice for themselves.

- **Fats** – oil, butter, margarine, and mayonnaise are approximately 120 calories per tablespoon. We all need some fat in our menu, but avoid using excessive amounts if you can. If you want the taste, only use a teaspoon for about 40 calories.

- **Sauces and dressings** – ask for these fat-laden delights to be served on the side. Use the fork method – lightly dip your fork into the dressing or sauce, and then pick up the lettuce or food. The small containers they use to serve dressing on the side usually have about four Tbsp. If they serve full-fat dressing, you are talking 280-400 calories for the dressing alone.

WHO WAS I KIDDING?

I remember when I was at my peak weight and I decided to order-in dinner for myself. Being very depressed (most likely over some guy!) I went through my mountain of delivery menus. I wasn't that hungry but needed the food to fill my emotional void. I decided on two slabs of ribs. I told the person taking the order that a friend was visiting. I am confident the person taking my order didn't care if I had a friend over or not — he just wanted my money!

Oh, the games we play to fool ourselves when we are in denial about how we eat!

EATING SALADS SUCCESSFULLY

When trying to lose weight, many choose salads as their go-to food. But salads aren't necessarily low calorie or low fat. Before we dive into dining out, let's set the record straight on salads. Some entrée salads served in restaurants have 800 to 1800+ calories, and the fat grams and sodium can be off the charts. Here are some tips on how to eat salads and not expand your waistline.

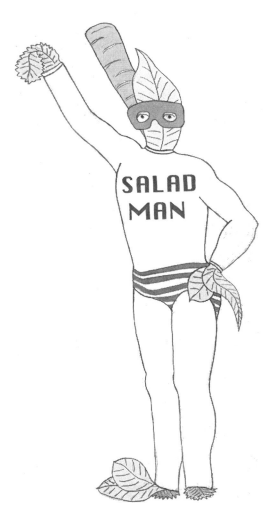

SALAD MAN

When you use lots of fruits and vegetables, you are adding vitamins and antioxidants. Add nuts and lean meats to your salad to make a great low-calorie, and highly nutritious meal.

FREE!

Up to 3 cups of the following veggies are basically calorie-free. We all need 5 to 9 servings of fruits and vegetables every day to meet the minimum daily requirements of the USDA...so eat up. Every five years, the Department of Health and Human Services (DHHS) and United States Department of Agriculture (USDA) jointly issue dietary guidelines for Americans, which are intended to guide policymakers, nutritionists, and nutrition education activities. In the latest report, which came out in January of 2011, the USDA recommended less sodium, less added sugar and less solid fat, and they promote filling half your plate with fruits and vegetables. By doing this at every meal, you will be eating more of what your body needs to be healthy and help you stay at your goal weight. The new guidelines stress a more plant-based diet. They encourage limiting the consumption of sugars and solid fats, and consuming less than 2300mg of sodium per day. These changes support Americans eating more produce so we can win the war against obesity.

Alfalfa sprouts
Artichokes
Asparagus
Broccoli
Carrots
Cauliflower
Cucumbers
Green beans
Hearts of Palm
Lettuce/salad greens
Mushrooms
Peppers
Pepperoncinis, Jalapenos, Sweet Peppers
Radishes
Snap Peas
Snow Peas
Sprouts
Tomatoes
Vegetable juice
Zucchini

WHAT TO DO:

- **Fruits** – sweeten your salad with fruit. A half cup of berries, citrus, apple or pear slices has approximately 40 calories.

- **Salad bars** – build your own for lots of variety. Avoid high-calorie or fatty toppings, mayonnaise, and oil-based side salads, such as pasta salad or coleslaw. Half of your plate should be raw or steamed vegetables.

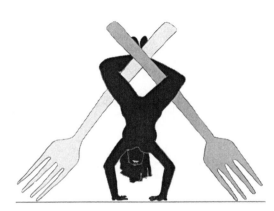

- **A little dip will do** – use the fork method. Dip your fork into the dressing, and then spear your salad to use minimal dressing, but still get the taste.

WHAT TO DO LESS OFTEN:

- **Meats and cheeses** – these have more calories than fruits and vegetables. The palm of your hand is one serving, or approximately 3 ounces.

- **Nuts** – great crunch appeal, but just a few will do. Limit your portion to a Tbsp.

- **Dress carefully!** – To lower the calories, dilute your dressing with lemon juice, vinegar, or water.

Freshly squeezed lemon or lime juice will tantalize your taste buds, and it has almost no calories. A 1/4 cup of salsa has about 25 calories, 2 tbsp of vinegar has about 15 calorie, 2 Tbsp of fat-free dressing has about 40–50 calories, 2 Tbsp of regular dressing has about 90 calories and 9g fat, and 2 Tbsp of creamy dressing has about 148 calories and 15.6g fat.

These calorie counts vary by brand. Read the label, when possible. If the label is not available, try to use the dressing sparingly.

- **Toppings you love** – please keep the portions small

  - Beans (garbanzo, kidney, black, etc.) – 1/4 cup = 60 calories, 0.5g fat, 2.5g fiber
  - Candied nuts – 2 Tbsp = 120 calories, 12g fat, 1g fiber
  - Cashews – 2 Tbsp = 160 calories, 13.3g fat, 0.9g fiber
  - Chopped egg – 1/4 cup = 55 calories, 4g fat, 0g fiber
  - Chow mein noodles – 1/4 cup = 130 calories, 5g fat, 0.3g fiber
  - Corn niblets – 1/4 cup = 40 calories, <0.5g fat, 1g fiber
  - Creamy coleslaw – 1/2 cup = 150 calories, 8g fat
  - Croutons – 1/2 cup = 75 calories, 3g fat, 0.5g fiber
  - Crumbled real bacon – 1 Tbsp = 60 calories, 5g fat
  - Imitation bacon bits – 2 Tbsp = 40 calories, 1.5g fat, 0.5g fiber
  - Dried fruit – 1/4 cup = 100 calories, <0.5g fat, 1g fiber
  - Full-fat cheeses – 1/4 cup = 100 calories, 8g fat, 0g fiber
  - Gorgonzola cheese crumbles – 2 Tbsp = 110 calories, 8g fat
  - Oil-marinated veggies – 1/3 cup = 100 calories
  - Olives – 2 Tbsp = 30 calories, 2.5g fat, 0g fiber
  - Pasta salad – 1/2 cup = 200 calories, 11g fat
  - Plain chunk tuna or chicken (no mayo) – 1/2 cup = 110 calories
  - Potato salad – 1/2 cup = 200 calories, 12g fat
  - Sunflower seeds – 2 Tbsp = 100 calories, 9g fat, 2g fiber
  - Sweetened dried cranberries – 1/3 cup = 138 calories, 0.5g fat, 3.7g fiber
  - Tortilla strips/ fried wontons – 1/3 cup = 100 calories, 5g fat, 0.5g fiber
  - Tuna or chicken salad with mayo – 1/2 cup = 250 calories, 20g fat

SALADS WITH A NAME....
FRIEND OR FOE?

Holy Caesar's ghost! A Caesar salad has romaine, parmesan cheese, croutons, and dressing.....but watch that dressing. Typically, the dressing is very high in calories. When you add the croutons and cheese, you have a license for disaster. Request the dressing on the side. That way, you can control how many calories you eat. Limit the croutons and cheese as they have a lot of fat and calories. Along with the dressing, these two items can make your salad go from 500 to 1500+ calories. If you add chicken or fish, make sure it is grilled, not fried.

Cobb salad – it will make you round ... unless you are careful. Cobb salad can be a meal in itself. But a Cobb salad can have 700 to 1800 calories, depending on what and how much is in it. The base is all lettuce, and as you learned in the previous section, lettuce is "free." The toppings are where you need to be careful. Special order this salad to eliminate excess calories and fat.

How to order a healthy Cobb salad:
• Make sure the chicken or fish is grilled, steamed or poached
• Ask for the bacon on the side so you can control the portion...or do without
• Remember that roquefort or blue cheese crumbles are 110 calories for 3 Tbsp - Ask for this cheese on the side to control the amount you use
• Ask for extra tomatoes
• Use avocado sparingly - An average-sized, whole avocado has 322 calories

Pass the chopsticks – Asian salads, like Chinese chicken salad, are quite popular. They commonly feature lettuce, Mandarin orange slices, wonton noodles, chicken, or sometimes, tuna or salmon. Some recipes add water chestnuts, bamboo shoots, ginger, peanuts, almonds, sesame seeds, and peppers. The dressing usually has soy sauce, peanut oil, sesame oil, chili oil, and seasonings.

How to order a healthy Chinese chicken salad:
- Hold the wontons (no need to add these fry-guys)
- Watch the dressing - the fork method lives on!
- Add just a few nuts
- Each almond is 10 calories, and each peanut is 4 calories
- Be careful, they add up quickly!

Fast food chains – everyone offers entrée salads. The trick is to order them "naked" and build from there. Caesars, Cobbs, or Asians can be ordered without the extras for around 100 calories … but that's not fun. Add the grilled chicken (not fried), and the average salad will be around 230 to 300 calories without the dressing. Go for the low-calorie dressing (most chains offer this option). Control the nuts and wontons. Thankfully, most fast food restaurants serve the toppings on the side.

CHINESE RESTAURANTS

While Chinese restaurant food is bad for your waistline and blood pressure (sodium contributes to hypertension) it does offer vegetable dishes and the kind of fat that's not bad for the heart. Popular Chinese restaurant meals can contain an entire day's worth of sodium and some contain two days' worth, according to a new analysis by the nonprofit Center for Science in the Public Interest. Food at Chinese restaurants is loaded with salt, calories, oil, noodles, and the batter used for deep frying. However, by knowing how to order, you can still enjoy this tasty cuisine and not jeopardize your weight loss goals.

WHAT TO DO:

- **Eat soup, but sparingly** – egg drop, wonton, and hot and sour soup have almost no calories or fat and will make you feel full. But be careful. They are extremely high in sodium, which can wreak havoc on your blood pressure. Also, when you add noodles or rice, you are adding calories, and the soups are no longer low-cal.

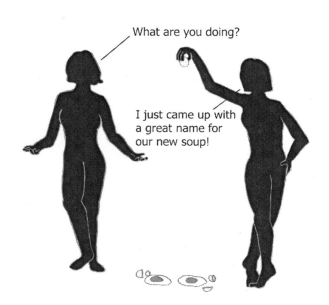

- **Pile on the veggies** – a staple in Chinese cuisine is vegetables, such as snow peas, carrots, green onions, and broccoli. Order them steamed with sauce on the side. Ask for these extra veggies to be added to your entrée, since they are nearly calorie-free!

- **Order chicken, tofu, or seafood** – these choices are always preferable to dishes with meat or noodles. Steamed or braised main dishes are better than dishes that are deep-fried, battered, or breaded.

- **Share** – since entrées average 700 to 1700 calories each, portion control rules! Share what is served, and fill your plate only one time so you are aware of how much you are eating.

- **Consider other Pan-Asian offerings** – some Chinese restaurants also serve sushi, which is a great alternative to traditional Chinese-American cuisine. Also, check out the Japanese restaurant section for the "411."

- **Use chopsticks** – even if you are not a master at using them, it will slow down the eating process.

- **Enjoy your good fortune** – fortune cookies are 30 calories each, with only a trace of fat.

WHAT TO DO LESS OFTEN:

- **Nix the fried options** – they are guaranteed to clog your arteries. Even if it is a fried *vegetable*, stay away! Egg rolls are fried, so order spring rolls (which are typically smaller and have a thinner wrap) for half the calories.

- **Separate the sauce** – order shrimp and broccoli or chicken with vegetables – or even a meat dish – but be sure to ask for the sauce on the side. A broken record? Yes, but it makes a difference. One Tbsp of soy sauce is only 10 calories but it has 920 mg of sodium in that one Tbsp. Almost half of your daily minimum requirement of sodium according to the USDA.

- **Say no to MSG** – studies have shown that the flavor enhancer monosodium glutamate (MSG), negatively affects every major system and organ in the body. What's more, adding MSG to foods has been shown to increase people's desire to eat faster and more frequently. The risk of being overweight was increased by 175% in people with a high intake of MSG, according to findings from a cross-sectional study published in the Nature journal *Obesity*. However, there are other studies that contradict this finding.

- **Rice is nice, but less is best** – you don't have to avoid rice; just limit your portion to one cup or less. To give you a visual, a cup – which is about 200 calories – is the size of a baseball or your fist. Brown rice is higher in fiber than white rice, and fried rice is the one to avoid at double the calories.

- **Dump the dumpling** – aka pot sticker. Pork dumplings are 85 calories, whereas vegetarian ones are 65. A 6-piece order is 400 to 500 calories, and you haven't even ordered your entrée! The best decision is to share an order so you can save calories for your entrée.

QUICK CALORIE KNOWLEDGE

Below are some fan favorite entrées. Since these entrées are usually very high in sodium and calories, it is wise to only eat half a portion.
- Beef and broccoli = 900 calories
- Chicken chow mein (varies but is lower calorie with rice than soft noodles) = 700 calories but if you add the crispy noodles, add 120+ calories
- Chicken with black bean sauce = 700 calories
- Ma po (Hunan) tofu (tofu and scallions) = 600 calories per order
- Moo goo gai pan (stir fried vegetables with chicken) = 600 calories
- Shrimp with garlic or lobster sauce = 700 calories
- Stir-fried mixed vegetables = 500 calories per order
- Szechuan shrimp = 700 calories

JAPANESE RESTAURANTS

Studies have proven that people eat up to 45% more food when served bigger helpings on large plates. And, as studies by Dr. Barbara Rolls (Pennsylvania State University) and Dr. Wansink (University of Illinois) and others suggest, faced with larger portions, people are likely to consume more, an effect, Dr. Rolls noted, that is not limited to people who are overweight.

In Japan, food is served on separate small plates and bowls instead of one big plate, resulting in less food consumed.

Sushi is normally served by the piece or the roll, which makes it easy to over-order. One way to cut calories is to bulk up your meal with other foods. Good choices are oshitashi (boiled spinach with soy sauce) or a small serving of edamame (lightly boiled soybeans). A 1/2-cup serving contains 127 calories, 6 grams of fat, and 4 grams of fiber.

WHAT TO DO:

- **Start with soup** – clear soups are filling, tasty, and low calorie. Miso soup is only around 50 calories per cup.

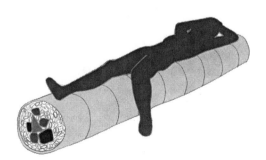

- **Don't be tempted by tempuras** – tempuras are very popular, but steer clear of them. Even the *vegetable* selections are deep fried.

- **Be sushi-savvy** – many sushi offerings are extremely low-calorie. One California roll is about 281 calories.

- **Nigiri is never a bad choice** – this oblong mound of rice, which is hand-pressed with a little wasabi and slice of fish, is an excellent addition to any entrée. Ask for light rice, to get lots of flavor, yet save a few calories.

- **Select sashimi** – this thinly sliced raw seafood is even better than nigiri. Since it has no rice, it averages about 25 to 50 calories per ounce.

- **Use chopsticks** – people usually eat slower when using chopsticks, even when they have expert skills.

WHAT TO DO LESS OFTEN:

- **Fatty fish?** – Salmon and eel are the two fattiest fishes, with 40% more calories than tuna, yellowtail, or scallops, so choose wisely. The up side is that they are good fats.
- **Spicy sauce** – it adds 50 – 70 calories per roll.
- **Sake** – at 39 calories an ounce, be thankful it is served in small cups as it doubles the calories of wine.
- **Rock 'n' roll** – Beware of rolls with special names, like Dragon, Rainbow, Tsunami, etc. They can be as high as 400 to 800 calories per roll. Avocado on any roll adds approximately 50 calories.

SPECIAL ROLL HINTS

The rule for "designer rolls" is, skip it or share it.
- "Crunch" is a clever way of saying "fried & fatty."
- "Dynamite" basically means "soaked in a sea of mayo."
- Spider rolls are as scary as the insect they are named after, full of calories and fat.

INDIAN RESTAURANTS

Focus on southern Indian food. By doing so, you'll get dishes made primarily from lentils, chick peas, and other legumes. Sauces will be based on zesty tropical flavors, rather than cream. Any Indian restaurant that features "masala dosa" in the menu is more likely to be serving southern food.

WHAT TO DO:

- **Check out the chicken** – try a chicken tikka entrée. Typically, this is pieces of boneless skinless chicken marinated in a varying array of flavors. This is not served in a sauce, it's just the chicken, at approximately 260 calories a serving. Also try chicken shashlik, which is really a kabob cooked in a tandoor. This dish is usually served with plain rice and some daal to keep it from being too dry.
- **Roti rocks** – often the roti or chapati breads are a far smaller serving size than the naan bread. A piece of roti or chapati with a 7" diameter = 60 calories. Roti is made from wheat flour or a whole wheat flour blend.
- **Savor a superb salad** – ask for a large serving. Indian salads are delicious, and they usually consist of a mix of cucumber, capsicum, cabbage, carrots, etc.
- **Try a terrific tandoori** – one chicken breast = 260 calories and 13g fat.

Best choices:

- Anything veggie in a tomato (not cream) sauce
- Bhaji or sag mushrooms
- Daal, aloo gobi, raita, and tandoori shrimp/chicken/fish are all fairly healthy

Rice rules – ask specifically for steamed rice and not just the rice they usually serve. The pilafs are almost always lightly fried in ghee before being steamed.

WHAT TO DO LESS OFTEN:

- **Steer clear** of fried appetizers like puri (fried bread), samosa, and pakoris.
- **Sidestep** traditional Indian yogurt dressings, which are usually made with whole milk yogurt. Try to find versions made with lower fat content.
- **Ghee**, a clarified butter used for basting, adds a lot to your fat intake, with 1 tsp = 45 calories.
- **Beware:**
  - Coconut milk or cream and all of the oil dishes.
  - Fried cheese appetizers.
  - Kheer, a rice pudding made with coconut milk, raisins and nuts can have over 500 calories.
  - Muglai (creamy curry sauce).
  - Naan = 1/4 (1.1 oz) = 79 calories (whole naan is 316 calories).
  - Paneer, kormas, rogan josh, masalas, and generally most of the curries used in the northern style dishes are staggeringly high in calories and fat.
  - Pilau has lots of oil.

Watch out for these words:

- Puri (fried bread)
- Muglai (cream sauce)
- Ghee (clarified butter)
- Khopre (coconut oil)

Think twice before ordering:

- Pork vindaloo curry- 620 calories
- Rogan josh: 500 calories- 30g fat
- Lamb pilaf: 520 calories- 35g fat
- Alu Ggosht kari- 600 calories

THAI RESTAURANTS

Eating Thai food is a wise decision because their dishes are mostly vegetables. An extra plus is that the food is cooked quickly, so the nutrients aren't lost.

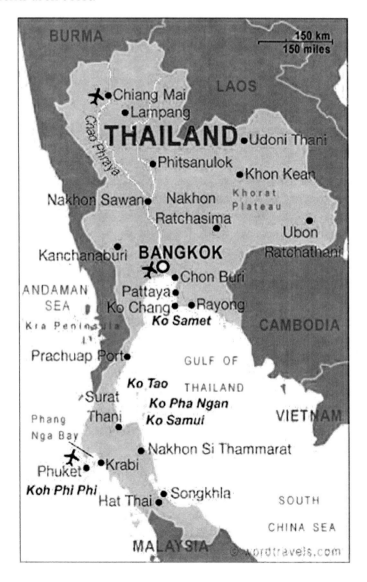

WHAT TO DO:

- **Stay with satay** – for many of us, satay is a favorite. Whether these delicious skewers are meat, chicken, or fish, they are low calorie – until you dip them in peanut sauce. Control your sauce; place 2 Tbsp of sauce on your dish for 80 calories.

- **Add some free calories** – hot chili peppers and lemongrass add some kick to your dish without adding calories.

- **Look for stir-fry** – best choices are white-meat chicken, tofu, and fish.

- **Search for steam** – appetizers like spring rolls and dumplings are steamed and low in calories.

- **Eat white or brown rice** – rice at 200 calories per cup is a popular offering at Thai restaurants. Opt for plain white or brown rice … or for a fun twist, try sticky rice. Flavored rices are about 380 calories per cup, while fried rice is a whopping 580 calories per cup.

QUICK CALORIE KNOWLEDGE

- Tom yum kung (hot-and-sour shrimp soup), 1 cup = about 100 calories
- Beef satay, 2 skewers without sauce = 250 calories
- Thai chicken with basil, 1 boneless, skinless breast, 3 oz. = about 225 calories
- Ginger chicken, 1 cup = about 350 calories
- Thai seafood salad, 2 cups = about 500 calories

WHAT TO DO LESS OFTEN:

- **Spare the sauces** – Thai restaurants cook a lot with coconut milk and peanut sauce, so be careful when ordering. Coconut is high in saturated fats and is not likely to help you keep your slim figure.

- **Say no to noodle dishes** – Pad Thai is a delicious and popular dish made with fried rice noodles. The sauce is so rich that I advise you eat only a small portion. A 1-cup serving is about 440 calories.

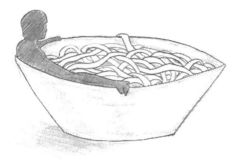

- **Limit the nuts? Oh nuts** – peanuts are another popular ingredient in Thai foods. They have good oils but still contain a lot of fat and calories, so it's best to limit them. Even 40 little peanuts are 170 calories.

- **What's a dinner without dessert?** – Thai sticky rice with mango and bananas in coconut cream are favorite desserts. However, coconut cream has 792 calories per cup, which makes these desserts very high in calories and fat. Fresh fruit is always your best bet.

MODERATION, PLEASE

- Kow neuw mamuang (mangoes with sticky rice) = 665 calories (just taste this one!)
- Mussaman beef curry, 1 cup = close to 1000 calories per serving
- Som loy geow (oranges in syrup) = 210 calories
- Thai beef salad, 1 cup = about 700 calories
- Thai coconut rice, 1 cup = 400 calories
- Thai coffee or tea, 1 cup = approximately 350 calories

MEXICAN RESTAURANTS

Mexican food packs a lethal punch in the fat and calorie department, so walk in with a plan. It is such a difficult cuisine to conquer, that we are starting with LESS OF THIS first!

WHAT TO DO LESS OFTEN:

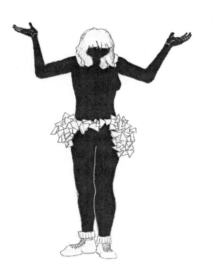

- **Chips on your hips?** – stop and think before grabbing your first chip. They are seemingly harmless, but they are addictive! You may never eat chips at home, but when served warm and crispy at your favorite Mexican eatery, it's hard to put on the brakes. The only healthy part is the salsa you are scooping up. If you do indulge, please count the chips out first – 12 to 15 chips = 140 calories

- **Burrito blast** – so popular, but so high in calories. Portion control is the plan. Consider eating half or even a third of a burrito.

  - Chicken Burrito = approximately 1100 calories
  - Vegetarian Burrito = approximately 1120 calories
  - Pork Burrito = approximately 1130 calories

- **Margaritaville** – beware of the calories that flavorful margaritas pack. They average 50 calories per ounce, and typical servings are 12 to 16 ounces. (See the What to Drink section for more "411.")

- **Say "cheese"?** – Most Mexican dishes are made with cheese, and they usually ring in at about 100 calories per ounce or slice.

Ask to go light on the cheese, then scrape off half of what is served.

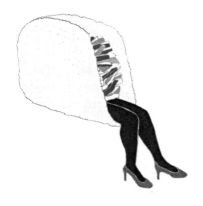

- **Tempting tortillas** – choose corn and whole wheat tortillas over flour tortillas, because they have fewer calories, less fat, and more fiber. Six-inch tortillas will help you keep your calorie intake under control.

- **Beware of the taco salad** – this dish sounds like it should be healthy but beware the cheese, sour cream, and guacamole. Most taco salads start at around 800 calories. *Holy enchilada!*

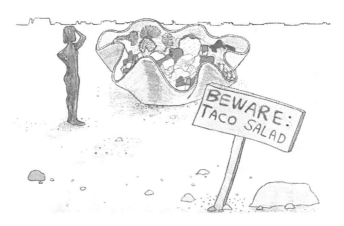

- **Enchiladas, chimichangas, burritos, and nachos, oh my!** – These choices are laden with fat. This is especially true when sour cream and guacamole are served as toppings, better known as "through your lips and to the hips!"

  - Enchilada = approximately 840 calories
  - Chimichangas = approximately 1,420 calories
  - Nachos = approximately 900 calories per serving

WHAT TO DO:

- **Go fish!** – Fish is always a great choice, since most fish is naturally low in calories and fat. Order it grilled or broiled with sauce on the side.

- **Fajitas are fabulous** – whether you order chicken, steak, or shrimp fajitas, ask for extra paper napkins so you can blot off any excess oil and save 50-100 calories. Use sour cream and avocado sparingly.

- **A great, meaty option** – most Mexican restaurants offer skirt steak, called carne asada. It is usually charbroiled and rubbed with spices or marinated. Ask for the sauce on the side, blot any excess oil, and limit your portion to 3 to 5 ounces (the size of your palm).

- **More beans, please** – these nutritious nuggets are loaded with fiber, complex carbohydrates (the good kind), protein, vitamins, and minerals. The best part: they are low in calories... about 210 per cup.

- **Love your salsa** – this delicious condiment is basically calorie-free, so enjoy! Much better than dipping your chips in guacamole, which is about 36 calories per Tbsp.

- **Dos Equis** – margaritas, move over. Instead, order a 12-ounce bottle, or two, of Mexican beer, at about 150 calories each.

Best Bets

Grilled seafood, lean meat, and poultry are excellent sources of protein, vitamins, and minerals. Choose dishes that have plenty of fresh veggies, including lettuce, tomatoes, and salsa. These foods are loaded with nutritional goodness, so load up on these foods to help fill you up. You can also request veggies in lieu of beans and rice.

BREAKFAST RESTAURANTS

If you are looking at this section, that's great news! That means you're going to eat the most important meal of the day instead of skipping it. Here's how you can make the best selections to start your day.

WHAT TO DO:

- **Egging you on to eat healthy** – The most popular breakfast option is eggs, but each egg yolk has 212 milligrams of cholesterol. Your daily intake of cholesterol should only be 300 milligrams. Best bet: *Order an egg white or egg substitute omelet.* To keep calories low, ask for the omelet to be cooked in non-stick spray instead of butter. Add as many veggies as you like, but try to avoid or limit cheeses and meats. Another healthy omelet option is to ask the server to use one whole egg and two egg whites.

- **Choose cereal, an excellent choice**! – Avoid sugary cereals and dive into steel-cut oatmeal. For cold cereal, read the Nutrition Facts to ensure each portion has at least 3 grams of fiber and under 200 calories per cup.

- **What's cereal without milk?** – Dry. Ha ha. Nonfat (skim) milk is your best choice. While 2% milk is okay, it's like drinking a cup of skim milk with a pat of butter in it. And whole milk is comparable to two pats of butter in your cup of skim milk! *Holy cow!* You could also use Greek yogurt instead of milk which adds lots of protein and makes you feel full for hours.

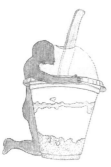

- **Go yogurt parfaits!** – The one at McDonald's is only 160 calories. Most parfaits are made with low fat yogurt, fruit, and granola. Be careful how much granola is included. It sounds healthy but often packs a lot of calories. Also watch the size of your parfait. Some are huge and, therefore, higher in calories (approximately 300 to 400 calories).

- **Boost your energy level** – order something you'll enjoy that gives you energy for the day. Egg whites and Greek yogurt are great choices for high protein.

WHAT TO DO LESS OFTEN:

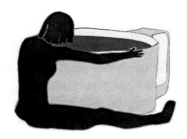

- **Limit caffeine** – the more caffeine you drink, the more you may feel the urge to eat. Too much caffeine can cause your body to work off your adrenaline versus burning fat cells. And remember, the less you add to your coffee, the better. You'll get a huge dose of unnecessary calories by ordering the fancy coffees served by your favorite barista at the corner coffee shop.

- **Let's talk juice** – did you know that one cup of orange juice is 112 calories and only 1/2 gram of fiber? On the other hand, if you eat an orange, it is only 85 calories and 4.3 grams of dietary fiber. It is always better to eat your fruit rather than drink it!

- **Go easy on the meat** – don't go overboard with bacon or sausage. Neither is high in calories, but they both have a lot of fat grams. Best bet: ask your friends to share one of their pieces so you won't feel deprived. Many restaurants offer turkey bacon or sausage which is lower in fat and calories. Other fan favorites are ham or Canadian bacon which should be limited to one piece.

- **Slow down on starches** – pancakes, French toast, waffles, or crepes are filling and delicious, especially with syrup and butter! Instead of ordering a full order for yourself, share a few bites with your friends, or ask for a side order to control the portion. And always remember to leave a third of what you are served on your plate.

- **Bread ... maybe** – consider your toppings and size. One slice of bread averages 70 calories; it's what you put on it that can get you in trouble. Your best bet is to just use jam or jelly, which is about 50 calories per Tbsp and no fat. Be careful when ordering bagels. Large ones are equivalent to the calories in 5 or 6 slices of bread!

STEAK RESTAURANTS

Plan ahead, and remember that portion control is essential in steak houses. Most steak houses are famous for their gigantic portions, which can easily be shared – especially side dishes and desserts. And since most steaks served in steakhouses are large, be sure to measure out 3 ounces for your meal (the size of your palm) and have the rest put in a doggie bag for another day. Even "petit" filets can be 8 to 10 ounces. Check the restaurant's website to learn your choices in advance. If they don't have a website, call first and ask for suggestions on what options would be best for watching your calories.

WHAT TO DO:

- **Spice things up** – a great way to make your meal more flavorful is to request peppercorn seasoning.

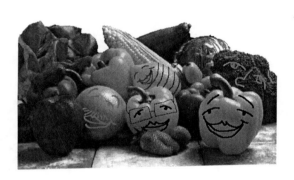

- **Pile on the veggies** – most steak restaurants offer steamed vegetables as an option for a side dish. You can eat as much of these as you like. Yeah, yeah, yeah. I know you want to top these beautiful steamed vegetables with hollandaise sauce. *Forget about it!*

- **Baked is beautiful** – potatoes and rice are staples at steak restaurants. The portions are usually insanely large, so limit your portion. Your best bet is to order a baked potato, which you can garnish with squeezed lemon, mustard, salsa, or green onion. Butter, sour cream, and shredded cheese are traditional toppers, but they pack a lot of fat and calories.

- **Not up for red meat?** – You can always find great fish selections – ask for the catch of the day for the freshest and tastiest option. You can also order a double shrimp cocktail as your entrée for a very low calorie meal.

- **End on a sweet note** – spend your calories wisely and order fruit or berries. If there is a dessert you crave, ask for several forks so everyone at the table will help you eat it. Try to limit yourself to 2 or 3 small bites so that you'll get the taste without feeling deprived. After the first couple of bites you don't taste it anyway, you are simply building a bicep.

- **Steak sauces** – add a little extra flavor, guilt-free. Steak sauces are only 12 to 15 calories per Tbsp.

WHAT TO DO LESS OFTEN:

- **Dig into a rib fest** – craving delicious BBQ ribs? Most steak houses serve them. The estimated calorie count for half a slab of ribs (1/2 pound with rub and marinade) is about 820 calories, 37g fat. I know, most folks eat a full rack, which is 1640 calories and 74g fat. Need I say more?

- **Beware of bread** – when the bread basket arrives, it's easy to eat a few slices with your cocktail before the meal order is taken. It is best to take one slice, then place the basket out of arm's reach. Remember, butter or oil will cost you about 100 to 120 calories per tablespoon. Most restaurant breads are warm and delicious without anything on them.

Which cut to be buff?

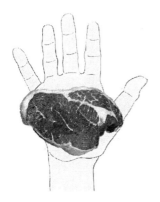

Always opt for the loin or round cuts at a restaurant or when purchasing meat for your home.

- Bison – 2g fat, 122 calories for a 3 oz serving, which is less than white meat chicken at 3g fat, 144 calories for 3 oz. Bison is similar to beef, but it tastes a little richer and sweeter.

- Sirloin – 6g fat, 150 calories for 3 ounces.
- Top round veal – 3g fat, 128 calories for 3 ounces.
- Other cuts like rib-eye, strip steak, or filet mignon are higher in fat content, so control your portion.
- If pork is your preference, choose leg cuts, such as ham, or loin.
- Boneless sirloin pork chops or top loin chops – 7g fat, 170 calories for 3 ounces.
- If you're a lamb lover – go for the shank half of the leg.
- Well-trimmed shank-half cuts have 5 to 6g fat and about 155 calories for 3 ounces.

SEAFOOD RESTAURANTS

I remember an old joke about the "see-food" diet: when I see it, I eat it!

Not a good idea. However, seafood is a brilliant choice when you are eating out or at home. Most nutrition researchers say eating seafood once or twice a week may be beneficial in preventing coronary heart disease. According to the Mayo Clinic website, doctors have long recognized that the unsaturated fats in fish, called omega-3 fatty acids, appear to reduce your risk of dying of heart disease. For many years, the American Heart Association has recommended that people eat fish rich in omega-3 fatty acids at least twice a week.

WHAT TO DO:

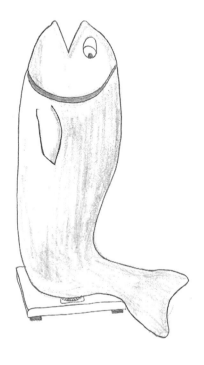

- **Bake, broil, grill, steam or poach** – there are so many good ways to order your seafood. Steer clear of the heavy creamy sauces, breading, and batters on the menu.

- **Crustaceans rock** – Lobster, crab legs, and shrimp are about 80-100 calories for 3 oz. The trouble begins when you dip it in butter. Butter is 120 calories per Tbsp. The butter coats your tongue, and you don't really enjoy the sweet taste of the fish. Squeeze lemon on your fish to enhance the flavors.

- **Go light** – rule of thumb is fish that is white are your best bets since they are all 100 calories or less for a 3 oz serving. That's about the size of the palm of your hand. Cod, flounder, halibut, monkfish, orange roughy, polack, rockfish, sea trout, tilapia, yellow fin tuna, sole and whiting are good choices.

- **Side dishes to be desired** – ask for steamed vegetables or a baked potato (the size of a computer mouse = 160 calories) and control the toppings. Use lemons to enhance the flavors of fish and your vegetables and potatoes as well.

WHAT TO DO LESS OFTEN:

- **Fat fish?** – Yes, some fish portions should be controlled. Fish high in fat are blue mussels, bluefish, mackerel, ocean perch, salmon, and shark.

- **Dipping disasters** – sauces can bring any meal down. Luckily seafood/cocktail sauce averages about 40 calories per Tbsp, but tartar sauce averages about 70 calories for one Tbsp. and is loaded with fat. Hence, the cocktail sauce is your best option, since it is fat-free. Another way to enhance fish is with a squeeze of lemon.

- **A tisket, a tasket, avoid the bread basket** – give yourself permission to have one slice of bread, and then strategically place the bread basket out of arm's reach. Or better yet, if it is okay with your dinner partner, ask to have it taken off the table entirely.

- **Delirious over dessert** – share one and have a taste or two so you don't feel deprived. Or order a bowl of berries, which are low-calorie and fat-free but still give you a sweet fix.

ITALIAN RESTAURANTS

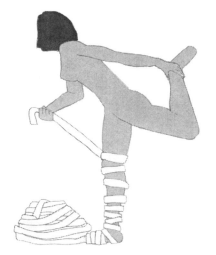

Pasta, pizza, olive oil, garlic bread, and Parmesan cheese come to mind immediately. Are you salivating yet? And if that wasn't enough to tantalize your taste buds, these restaurants typically serve portions that are big enough to serve a family of six. By following some simple guidelines, you will be able to enjoy the great flavors of Italian cuisine without hating yourself the next day.

PASTA WORKOUT

WHAT TO DO:

- **Go for grilled** – select an entrée that offers grilled fish, meat or chicken with a side of pasta, instead of an entrée that is pasta and sauce only.

- **Portion your pasta** – pasta has a low glycemic index, so it's a good choice because it keeps blood sugar levels steady. This makes between-meal sugar cravings less likely. It doesn't matter which pasta you choose as long as they are whole grain (they all average about 200 calories per cup), but pick your sauce wisely.

- **Make it veggie time** – I highly recommend ordering a side of steamed broccoli, asparagus, or the restaurant's vegetable of the day.

- **Pass the pizza, please** – many Italian restaurants make small pizzas that are about 12 inches in diameter and baked with a thin

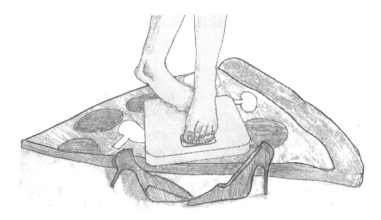

crust. Control your portions, and you can safely eat two slices from a small or medium pizza and only spend about 300-350 calories. One slice of deep dish pizza has anywhere from 350-580 calories. Most pizza restaurants have a full menu with salads, entrées, and sandwiches. If two slices of pizza are not enough for you, order a veggie soup or salad to eat first and ask for dressing on the side. Ask for whole grain crust, it is always better than white.

- **Dealing with dessert** – when it comes to dessert, tiramisu, cannoli, and gelato are all delicious. They are also loaded with calories, so order your favorite and share it with everyone at the table. If you want your own dessert, go for the berries or a fruit cup. Many Italian restaurants offer flavorful sorbets that are only 140 to 180 calories per scoop and low in fat.

WHAT TO DO LESS OFTEN:

- **Ease up on antipasto** – antipasto is a wonderful appetizer made up of lots of veggies, meats, and cheeses. Even if it's all veggies, beware of the oil in the marinade. If you choose this dish, use a slice of bread to blot off any excess oil. Then leave that slice of bread on the plate for the busboy to take away.

- **Brush up on bruschetta knowledge** – bruschetta seems like an innocent choice made with chopped, seasoned tomatoes on top of bread slices. But once again, it's about the oil they pour on top. At 120 calories per Tbsp, olive oil can pack a punch. Some restaurants top their bruschetta with crumbled cheese. Ask for the cheese on the side to control the calories. Each piece of bruschetta, depending on the size and ingredients, is about 130-245 calories.

- **Don't ham it up** – Italian deli meats like prosciutto and other hams are not just high in fat, but also high in salt. In other words, your rings are going to be tight the next morning!

- **Cheese, please?** – ask for less cheese on your pasta (or no cheese at all), and request that your meat toppings be cut in half. You can always add lots of veggies. Topping off anything with shredded Parmesan is okay if you limit the portion. It is only 25 calories per Tbsp.

- **Avoid cream-based, cheesy, and oily sauces** – go for tomato-based sauces with a lower fat and calorie count.

GREEK RESTAURANTS

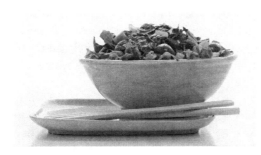

Greek food is amazing. With a healthy concentration of fresh fruits, vegetables, grains, and legumes, you can select from many tasty meat and seafood options. Generally, however, the calories in Greek food are not known to be especially low. As with any cuisine, don't forget when eating out to focus on your friends and remember that sharing your dinner is a great plan.

WHAT TO DO:

- **Begin with a healthy starter** – baba ghanoush (eggplant appetizer) is a tasty treat at only 50 calories for 2 Tbsp. Other good starters are grilled veggies or cold fish such as raw oysters, clams, or shrimp.

- **Devour delectable dips** – try the yogurt and cucumber dip (tzatziki) at 20 calories per Tbsp. Hummus, which is high in fiber, comes in at about 25 to 40 calories per Tbsp. Use veggies for dipping instead of the oil-laden pita chips.

- **Make it meze** – this is a traditional Greek starter of hot and cold appetizers, which are piled in the middle of the table so everyone can help themselves. This means you can have as much or as little as you want. Stick to grilled veggies, or tzatziki with veggies if you don't want to pile on the calories.

- **Go for the Greek salad** – Greek salads have gone main stream – and we are so glad they did! Limit the olives (which are low calorie but high fat) and the feta cheese, which is lower in fat and calories than a lot of other cheeses. And ask for the dressing on the side so your salad isn't sitting in a pool of oil.

- **Select souvlaki** – this popular dish is made up of grilled meats (usually pork or chicken) and veggies on skewers which is portion controlled and healthy. They can also be served on a pita with sauces or as an entrée with sides like rice pilaf or potatoes.

- **Load up on veggies** – many Greek meals consist of delicious Mediterranean vegetables – the basis of a healthy meal.

WHAT TO DO LESS OFTEN:

- **Extra virgin olive oil (EVOO) … it's a love/hate relationship** – Greek foods are prepared with a lot of olive oil, which is heart-healthy when used in small portions (particularly extra-virgin olive oil). But beware of dishes swimming in EVOO, which is 120 calories per Tbsp.

- **Minimize the moussaka** – this popular dish is particularly delicious because of all the fatty, rich, and cheesy ingredients. Treat it like a dessert, and take a bite or two of someone else's portion.

- **Sliver of spanakopita only** – this spinach and cheese pie is delicious, but it can have as many calories as moussaka depending on the portion size. Again, just have a few bites.

- **Dole out the dolmades** – an entrée-size (4 pieces is 12 oz) serving of this traditional dish (grape leaves filled with meat and rice) = 540 calories. Try sampling instead of having the whole entrée.

- **No-go the gyro!** – the gyro is a pita-bread sandwich filled with a molded mixture of seasoned beef and lamb roasted on a vertical spit. The 5 ounces of meat in a typical sandwich delivers 44 grams of fat, including a whole day's worth of artery-clogging fat (20 grams). The 760-calorie sandwich also provides close to an entire day's worth of sodium.

- **Beware of the baklava** – yes, it's tempting, but baklava is made with chopped walnuts and almonds, cinnamon, cloves, and phyllo dough, all drizzled with honey. If you select this delicious pastry, have only one or two bites.

FRENCH RESTAURANTS - BON APPETIT!

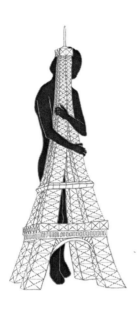

The French take pride in their cooking, as well as the taste and appearance of their food. French chefs use lots of cream, butter, oil, and wine in their cooking so it's important to choose carefully from the menu. Ask about any ingredients you aren't sure about, and order all sauces and dressings on the side. Follow these strategies for some ooh-la-la French meals – minus the guilt!

WHAT TO DO:

- **Raw ... it's the way to go!** – oysters and snails are divine when eaten sans sauce. Oysters are the best, they only need a squeeze of lemon, horseradish and/or hot sauce and are only 60 calories for 8 oysters! And mussels are only 136 calories per three ounce serving.

- **Go fish?** – obviously grilled fish is your best selection. Other preparations can be pared down by asking for sauces on the side. Taking half of it home for another meal or sharing an entrée is always a good option for minimizing the calories in this delicious cuisine.

- **Jump on the frog legs** – this traditional French dish is only about 130 calories for 4 oz but watch the butter-dipping ritual, which can add inches to *your* legs.

- **Do dessert!** – the best choices for dessert in a French bistro are around 270 to 350 calories per serving depending on the recipe: Crème caramel is lowest, followed by chocolate mousse and crème brûlée. Fruit or berries are always the best option. Some restaurants will offer meringues which are very low calorie.

- **Cheese, please** – since French pastries are very high in calories (220 to 600 per serving), you might want to follow the age-old tradition of having cheese after your meal. You'll consume 115 calories for an ounce of hard cheese, 90 calories for an ounce of brie or Camembert, and 50 to 80 calories per ounce for goat cheese. Not too many crackers, and you will keep your calories in check.

WHAT TO DO LESS OFTEN:

- **Enjoy your wine – sparingly!** – wine is a major food group in France. One of my clients found success in saving her wine for dessert. A glass is only 20 calories per ounce, and a whole bottle is about 500 calories.

- **Other starters** – French onion soup, which is about 400+ calories per serving, is a lot for a starter. Another famous preparation is escargots (snails), which involves sauce made with butter, parsley, garlic, and spices at 300 calories per serving. Not light at all. Try one from someone else's plate.

- **Bread yes, croissant no** – think twice before sinking your teeth into a light and flaky croissant at 350 calories. Instead, choose a small piece of French bread at 55 calories.

- **Don't break the law** – for a while it was against the law in Chicago to serve foie gras (duck or goose liver), but if you can still order this divine dish, chose it as your appetizer and enjoy a small portion. 1 oz = 131 calories and 12.4 grams of fat. One Tbsp = 65 calories.

Can't find your entrée? Look under the sauce.

To keep your waistline narrow, ask for the sauce on the side. Great French entrées are:

- Grilled dover sole = 220 calories
- Grilled trout = 250 calories
- Coq au vin = 585 calories
- Steak au poivre = 490 calories
- Steak with béarnaise sauce = 575 calories
- Beef bourguignon = 635 calories
- Duck in orange sauce = 840 calories

Did you say French pastry? – here's the skinny on how to order your last course.

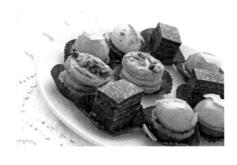

- From crepe suzettes to fruit tarts, your calories will range from 400 to 500 calories per serving. Please share.

- **Going for the big one?** – order profiteroles at 600+ calories per serving and share it. Between the pastry, the sauce, and the ice cream, you will be in sugar shock for days.

- **Decadent desserts** – to be shared and enjoyed with an espresso after dinner.

  - Crème caramel = 215 calories
  - Crème brûlée = 350 calories
  - Crepe suzette = 400 calories
  - Tarte tatin = 525 calories
  - Profiteroles = 600 calories
  - Meringues = average about 20-30 calories each

FAST FOOD RESTAURANTS

Always do your homework and get to know your favorite fast food restaurant's nutritional information. Most will provide you with a nutritional fact sheet when asked. You also can look up information online before you go. Many of the national chains are posting their calorie counts on their menu boards which is wonderful in helping us make smart decisions.

WHAT TO DO:

- **Breakfast: keep it cold** – many fast food restaurants offer cold cereal with non-fat milk – a quick, easy, and calorie-controlled choice – whereas some other choices have as many as 1500 calories. Check the nutritional breakdown for the most up-to-date information. Even if some breakfast sandwiches are only 300 to 400 calories, they still have enough fat grams for your entire day.

- **Burger madness** – if you are hankering for a hamburger, order the small burger or cheeseburger rather than a quarter-pounder or other "named" burgers that are loaded with extras like bacon, special sauce, and cheese. A downsized version will save you 200 to 500 calories and 20 to 30 grams of fat.

- **Salads-only some will do** – depending on the ingredients, some salads are very low calorie when served with a fat-free or low-cal dressing. Check the nutrition facts, read labels, then make the best choice. Choose a dressing that doesn't exceed 50 calories for 2 Tbsp.

- **Choose chicken** – chicken is usually a better option than red meat, but be sure to go for the grilled version and nix anything breaded or fried.

WHAT TO DO LESS OFTEN:

- **Bag the bagel.** Would you eat 4 to 6 slices of toast for breakfast? Heck no! The large bagels range from 320 to 500 calories each. Regular cream cheese adds 50 calories per Tbsp and you will add 30 calories per Tbsp for the light version—and definitely skip the bagel sandwiches. If you crave a bagel, eat half and save the other half for tomorrow's breakfast. Or, you can save 50-60 calories by scooping out the bread from the inside of the bagel.

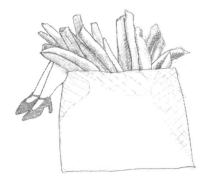

- **Enter the no fry-zone** – if you must have French fries, ask for the small size. Then, share your fries with friends or eat half and pitch the rest. Your best bet will always be the grilled offerings instead of fried foods.

- **Beverages? So many empty choices** – this is one place where you have lots of options… lots of empty calorie options. Avoid juices, regular soda pop, or high-calorie coffee drinks. Opt for the diet pop or, better yet, buy a bottle of water. (You can also ask for a cup of water, and it's free!)

- **Best bet: kids' meals!** – Why not? We are all kids at heart. Many fast-food restaurants now have options with fruit instead of fries, and you can get a whole meal for the same calories as some of the "grown-up" sandwiches.

DELIS AND SANDWICH SHOPS

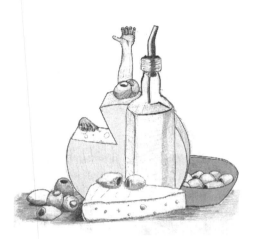

These popular eateries offer foods that are tasty, filling, and easy to eat on the run. The danger zones are the condiments, the bread, and the cheeses.

WHAT TO DO:

- **"Skinny" your sandwich** – some chains let you "skinny" your sandwich by tearing away the bread from the inside of the roll, thus throwing away about 50 to 60 calories. To accomplish a similar result, order your sandwich open-faced. Or eat half of the sandwich and save the remainder for the next day, or pitch it.

- **Select healthy and slice 'em thin** – your best choices are lean roast beef slices (about 40 to 50 calories each), ham slices (about 50 calories each), and turkey slices (around 20 to 40 calories each). Beware of high-fat meats like corned beef and pastrami, as they're packed with both fat and sodium.

- **Lox... the great bagel protector** – ordering lox is a great choice, as smoked salmon is only about 33 calories per ounce. It's the cream cheese and bagel that will get you in trouble. Eat only half the bagel, and top it with a limited smear of low-fat cream cheese, tomatoes, and lettuce. Stay away from herring and other smoked or pickled fish, which are high in fat and sodium.

- **Wrap-o-rama** – sandwiches in the form of wraps are the hot new item. If this is served large, only eat half and save the other half for the next day. Always be sure to keep the condiments and cheese to a minimum. The tortilla wrap alone ranges from 100 to 350 calories, depending on the size and ingredients.

- **Super soups.** A great choice, when you choose broth-based soups and avoid the creamy ones. Chicken soup is not only low calorie, but is also medicinal... ask any Jewish mother. Great choices are:

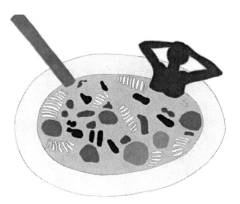

  - Chicken noodle soup
  - Chicken matzo ball soup
  - Cabbage soup
  - Vegetable soup
  - Mushroom barley
  - Vegetable soup
  - Beet borsht, only 75 calories per cup (sour cream on the side)
  - Split pea

- **Gefilte fish ranks high on the list of non-swimmers** – 3 oz. = 75 calories, not bad. For great flavor and no calories, top it with "crane" (horseradish).

- **Tried 'n' true toppings** – toppings that you can enjoy without limit:
  - Mustard – great flavor and most brands have no fat.
  - Salsa – another great condiment to add flavor without any calories.
  - Vegetables – use them to bulk up any sandwich for more flavor and crunch.
  - Peppers – a good way to spice up your sub without hurting anything but your tongue

WHAT TO DO LESS OFTEN:

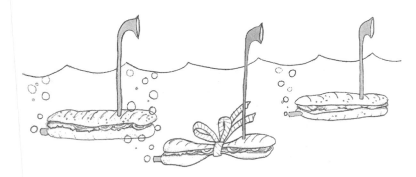

- **Silly sides** – most side dishes are high-fat and high-calorie. If you are craving potato salad or coleslaw, order the smallest portion available, take a couple of bites, and either share or throw out the rest.

- **More silly sides ... chips and fries** – go for the small bag of baked chips versus the deep fried variety. A small bag of baked chips is only 130 calories. If fries are your guilty pleasure, then count out 5-10 of those little fry guys.

- **Troublesome toppings** – for calorie control and health benefits, either avoid these toppings or use them sparingly:
    - Cheese = averages about 100 calories per slice
    - Oil, butter, and mayo = average about 100–120 calories per Tbsp
    - Pickles = low in calories, but high in sodium
    - Olives = low calorie, but very high in fat

- ***Tradition!*** Other traditional foods worth ordering at the neighborhood deli are great in small portions.
    - Blintzes = about 100 calories each; top with applesauce or 1 Tbsp of sour cream
    - Matzo balls (aka knaidlach) = 70 calories for the big ones, 1" ball = 25 calories
    - Noodle kugel = about 220 calories for a small piece
    - Spinach and cheese knish = approximately 100 calories for a small piece

WHAT TO DRINK:
NONALCOHOLIC BEVERAGES

The best choice is always water. Add a slice of lemon, lime, or cucumber, or a splash of juice for flavor.

WHAT TO DO:

- **Coffee and tea – they're calorie-free!** – watch out for the add-ons. Cream is 20 calories per Tbsp, and sugar is 16 calories per teaspoon. It doesn't sound like much, but it does add up if you drink multiple cups.

- **Lighten up, Elsie!** – if you are into fancy coffee drinks, always request non-fat milk to cut calories. For example, a 12-ounce non-fat latte is only 90 calories; with whole milk, it's 200 calories. Size is also a factor. A 16-ounce grande non-fat latte is 160 calories. And please, forget the whipped cream!

WHAT TO DO LESS OFTEN:

- **Be a sport ... but be careful of their drink** – sport drinks have taken over whole sections in grocery stores. They are very popular, but they are also high in calories (50 calories per 8 oz serving; some bottles have 4 servings). On the up side, they are great for replacing your electrolytes. If you have worked out intensely and need one, control your portion. Or opt for the new "light" sports drinks on the market today at 25 calories per 8 oz serving. There are also waters that have electrolytes and no calories.

- **Do you say "soda" or do you say "pop"?** – soda pop is loaded with calories. One serving averages about 12 calories per ounce, which is about 144 calories per 12 oz can. Diet pop is a better choice, but you are always better off with a glass of water.

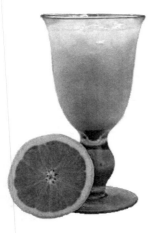

- **Juices ... only so-so** – they are great for nutrients, high in calories, and low in fiber. If you want juice, limit the portion size. Or better yet, eat a piece of fruit – an 8 oz glass of orange juice is 112 calories, and a large orange is only 86 calories with 4 1/2 grams of fiber.

WHAT TO DRINK: COCKTAILS

Cocktails are a big part of being social, and just because you are watching your waistline doesn't mean you can't socialize! Once again, it is all about portion control and smart choices. Most alcoholic drinks contain no fat, but alcohol has high calorie content.

Thinking back, I have always been a lightweight or cheap date, so I wasn't challenged by drinking too much when I was overweight. That's a good thing. The benefits of not having more than one or two drinks during an evening are:

- not saying things "under the influence,"
- not waking up the next day with a hangover, and, most importantly,
- not having to suffer a beer belly, which lasts *a lot* longer than your drink does!

Trust me, you can still have fun. Volunteer to be the designated driver, and everyone wins.

Drink This Way (It would be irresponsible to say "More of This" or WHAT TO DO)

You know the old adage, "One martini, two martinis, three martinis, floor!"

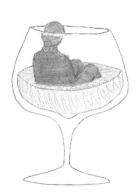

Please be careful, and don't drink and drive.

- **Wine is wonderful** – wine (or champagne) is about 20 calories per ounce, so a 6-ounce glass of wine is about 120 calories. You could share a bottle, which averages about 500 calories.

- **"Lite" is right** – when it comes to beer, there are two ways to go. Light beers are around 100 calories, and regular beer is about 145 calories. It doesn't sound like a lot, but if you have more than one, the calories add up quickly. Some light beers on the market have only 64 calories.

- **Go neat or on-the-rocks** – cocktails made with distilled liquor (e.g., 80-proof scotch, bourbon, vodka, gin, or rum) average about 64 calories per ounce. You wouldn't be happy if your bartender only poured one ounce, so I would guess you are usually being served a jigger, which is about 128 calories of alcohol. Drink it on the rocks, with water or club soda to avoid adding calories. *Martinis rule here – you get an immediate buzz and don't need a second drink. But watch the driving.*

- **Faux cocktail** – if you want something that tastes special with no calories, order a club soda with bitters garnished with a lemon or lime. It looks like a cocktail, it tastes like a cocktail, and it's calorie-free!

Avoid Drinking This Way

- **Visit the tropics, don't drink them** – tropical drinks such as margaritas and pina coladas are about 50 calories per ounce. Because they are usually served in humongous glasses, they end up at 600 to 800 calories per drink! Ask the person you are with for a sip of theirs, and order something with fewer calories for yourself. When trying to lose weight, it's best to avoid these drinks like the plague. If you're maintaining your weight, it's okay to indulge on special occasions.

- **No mixing allowed** – mixers add up to 100 to 150 more calories, depending on the size of the glass. Juices, cola, tonic, and other sugary pops should be avoided.

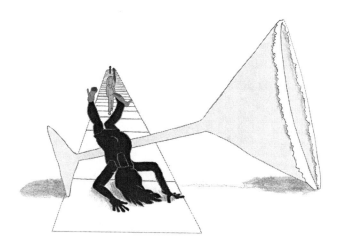

- **After-dinner drinks** – another term for sugary liqueurs. These drinks should be avoided or at least limited to one. They are high in calories and can trigger your sweet tooth. And on top of a long evening, they will seal the deal for a hangover.

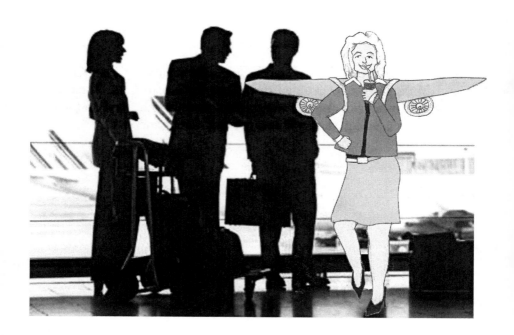

SECTION TWO:

Eating when traveling

A Traveler's Reality

I don't know what came over me, but the minute my bags were checked, I felt I had a license to eat. When I went on pleasure trips, I got this mentality because it seemed acceptable to take a vacation from everything – including my healthy eating plan. On business trips, I justified the license to eat because, after all, didn't I deserve a little extra pleasure as a reward for working so hard?

Those were the days before I took control of my eating. We all do it, but there are ways to travel and not overindulge. No matter how well you can justify that big fat muffin or the huge aromatic cinnamon roll at the airport or the pralines in New Orleans, or a heaping helping of biscuits and gravy in Nashville – at the end of the day, it isn't worth the calories.

EATING AT AIRPORTS

As always, start with a plan. While it's best to eat at home before your flight, the reality is we are usually rushing out the door, and we have to make the most of what the airport has to offer.

Start with being selective. No matter how hungry you are, don't commit to the first food stand you encounter. If there's a directory of restaurants, check it out and go to the one that sounds the healthiest. Better yet, if you have the time, walk around the airport and log a lot of steps looking for the best place. Consider whether you want to select from a kiosk with sandwich and salad offerings or a sit-down restaurant that serves full meals.

WHAT TO DO:

- **Healthy starts** – order cereal with yogurt or low-fat milk. If there's a McDonald's, consider a parfait for only 160 calories. A small egg sandwich can be very filling. To make this meal healthier, hold the high-calorie, high-fat add-ons like cheese, bacon, sausage, or butter. One more way to cut back on calories: toss half the bread.

- **Your coffee "fix"** – if it's coffee you crave or caffeine you need, treat yourself to a plain old cup of Joe. For something fancier, go for a small or medium non-fat latte or cappuccino – without the whipped cream. Beware of the extra-large whipped cream coffee drinks that contain the calories and fat of a whole meal.

- **Sensible salad** – limit or omit fatty add-ons like cheese, bacon, avocados, fatty meats, and fried toppings such as croutons. Check out pages 18-19 for the skinny on salads.

- **Open-faced is best** – if you're going for a sandwich, cut calories by throwing away half the bread or, better yet, half the sandwich. For more great tips on how to order a sandwich, look at the deli section on pages 52-54.

- **Recharge with H_2O** – always have a bottle of water with you so you can refill it and keep hydrating. It gives you a feeling of being full. You will need to buy this after you go through security since they will make you pitch any liquids you have with you.

WHAT TO DO LESS OFTEN:

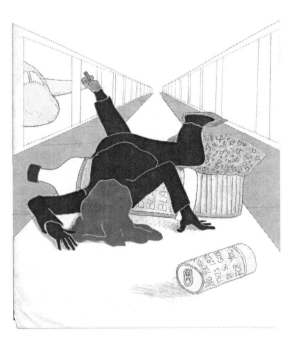

- **Bounce the bagel** – big bagels are high in calories, especially those with seeds. Eat half (get whole grain, if possible), and eat it plain or with a dab of light cream cheese or jelly. Peanut butter is a great source of protein, and 1 Tbsp adds 90 calories. To cut calories, use a teaspoon instead.

- **Don't get twisted** – if you want a large pretzel, ask for one made without butter. The lowest calorie options are the original, garlic or jalapeno pretzels, which are about 270 to 320 calories each. The others can be as high as 510 calories...*now that's twisted!*

- **Craving a snack?** – reach for a yogurt or fresh fruit. Bananas, apples, and oranges are frequently sold at concession stands, and they are much better than cookies, potato chips, or candy bars. Nuts and trail mix aren't all bad, since they offer great protein and good fats. Portion control rules, since they are high-calorie and full of salt. Packages of 100-calorie crackers are easy to carry when traveling. Read the labels on 100-calorie packs, since some types can be very high in fat. Here are some good options you can find on the concourse:

- Grilled chicken sandwich (without mayo or creamy condiments)
- Bean burrito (if it's huge, eat half; share the other half or pitch it)
- Popcorn (unbuttered)
- Turkey sandwich (without mayo)
- One slice of thin cheese pizza
- Smoothies – check the nutrient facts before you order so you know the calorie and fat counts.
- Salad greens and raw veggies topped with grilled lean meat or seafood – ask for light or fat-free salad dressing served on the side.

TAKING A LONG FLIGHT

When it's time for a longer trip, always plan ahead and carry enough food so you have snacks available from when you arrive at the airport until you arrive safely at your destination. Bring books, crossword puzzles, magazines, DVDs, or your laptop to keep yourself busy and keep your mind off food.

WHAT TO DO:

- **Stay hydrated** – bring big bottles of water and drink them on your flight. You will feel much better when you land. Airports will not allow liquids to go through the security, but you can purchase bottles of water after you have passed the security checkpoints.

- **Airline aerobics** – *get up!* Move around the cabin, walk the aisles, do squats, deep knee bends etc. You will feel much better when you arrive at your destination. A friend of mine told me her husband walked the aisles all the way home from Australia to the states because he couldn't sit still. Great exercise, huh?

- **Do the math** – on long-distance flights, there can be a big difference in time zones. Combine the first two days of your trip and treat it like one 2500-calorie day (men should eat 3400 calories). It makes it easier to calculate what you are eating during this transitional time.

- **Packin' and snackin'** – don't forget to pack napkins or moist towels. Here are some snacks that travel well:
  - 10 almonds = 100 calories
  - 1 box of raisins (1/4 cup) = 130 calories
  - Pretzels = 100 calories portion (check package for measurement)
  - Dry cereal = 100 calories worth of cereal to eat as a snack dry or request skim milk from the flight attendant.

WHAT TO DO LESS OFTEN:

- **Nix the onboard airplane snacks** – those cute little packets of nuts are not so bad if you have just one. The packets of nuts served on Southwest airlines are 70 calories each and the pretzels are 50 calories per pack. On longer flights they offer cookies and other tempting treats, but do yourself a favor and avoid the ones with sugar and bad carbs. Instead, bring fresh fruit, veggies, or a sandwich to satisfy your hunger.

- **Meals onboard, plan ahead** – call the airline in advance to inquire about the food service on your flight. This way, you'll be able to supplement what they offer with your own snacks. When you call at least 48 hours in advance, you can order from a variety of special meals to meet your dietary needs. For example, if you are diabetic, vegetarian, or kosher you can order the kind of meal you need. Obviously this only applies to long flights where they still serve meals.

- **Hold the cocktails** – abstaining from alcoholic beverages in flight (and drinking lots of water instead) is both a physical and a mental remedy. It helps to offset dehydration and promotes mental clarity. Why not save these calories until you get to your destination, especially if it's a gorgeous, beachfront resort?

EATING ON BUSINESS TRIPS

It bears repeating. Being on the road for business is not a license to eat anything and everything. Like any other day, you must start your day with a plan. Knowing what you are going to eat will ensure a successful eating day.

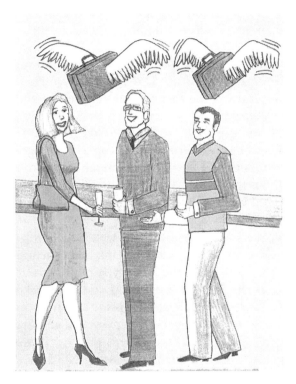

Long days – pack emergency foods for when you get caught in a meeting and the only option is junk food. Good options are raisins, tuna in a pouch, peanut butter, graham crackers, rice cakes, 100-calorie packs, protein bars etc.

An apple a day – find a local grocery store when you arrive at your destination and buy fresh produce and water to put in your hotel fridge to create a healthy environment. You can ask the hotel to empty your mini-bar for this purpose. You can also find fresh fruit at your corner coffee shop.

Breakfast options – instead of eating at the buffet, take control of your eating and order off the menu. My personal favorites are egg white omelets, oatmeal, or any high-fiber cereal with skim milk. Limit or avoid the high-fat breakfast meats and cheesy additions.

Time for lunch – whether you eat lunch in or out, eat for energy and a small waistline. This can best be done when you eat 3 to 5 oz of protein, grilled or broiled. Avoid foods that will make you drag in the afternoon, such as sugary desserts or fatty French fries. Eat your sandwich with one slice of whole grain bread. If you opt for a salad, order the dressing on the side and request their low-cal dressing.

Snack attack – to be prepared, stop at a convenience or grocery store and stock up on healthy snacks. Your best bets will be raw veggies, fresh fruit, low-fat or fat-free yogurt, V8 juice, rice cakes, etc.

Happy Hour – are you drinking after work to bond with a client or co-worker on the road? Sounds like fun. Did you know you can go out with the group and not drink the rest of your calories for the day? If you choose to have one or two cocktails, that is fine. But then switch to water, either flat or sparkling. Club soda with lime or lemon looks like a cocktail and has no calories. You can ask the bartender to add a splash of bitters to add flavor. Remember, it is about the conversation and not about the drinks! Check pages 57-59 for the "411" on cocktails.

Dinners done right – dinners with clients can create a huge temptation to overeat. The meal is all about building your relationship with your client. You don't have to order the same type of meal your client orders. You can go to the best of restaurants and still make smart food choices. Check the restaurant's website prior to dinner to see what they have on their menu. When you arrive, you will already know what you are ordering, and it will be easier to pass on those tempting specials. You can also choose healthy restaurants, and your clients will probably appreciate it.

SECTION THREE:

Eating at Work

WHAT TO EAT AT WORK

Taking control is the first step to healthy eating at work, the place where we spend the majority of our time. To successfully conquer this challenge, plan what your meals and snacks will be for the day. Keep fruit and cut vegetables at your desk to ensure healthy eating. Relax and take your time when you eat. If possible, don't eat meals at your desk. Instead, go to the lunch room or outside of the office. Food is much more satisfying when you have the time to focus on what you are eating, instead of inhaling it between talking on the phone and answering emails at your desk.

Breaking Bread with Others

Control your portions and order according to your plan for the day. Don't let your co-workers or clients influence how you order. This is not an eating competition. Instead, it is a time to have enjoyable conversation or to discuss business matters.

Whether ordering in for lunch or going out, always look for the following magic words:
- Grilled
- Baked
- Broiled
- Garden fresh
- Roasted
- Poached
- Steamed

Too Busy for Lunch

"Just bring me back something!" – did someone say they were going to Taco Bell? McDonald's? Doesn't matter where, this type of knee-jerk reaction is a good way to add many high-fat, high-sodium foods to your diet. If this is the only way you can get some lunch, go to the website of choice and order wisely. Smaller sandwiches give you the flavor without all the extra calories.

Coffee in lieu of lunch? – with no time to eat and lots of fancy coffee shops around, it is one more place to chalk up a load of calories and caffeine while you lighten your wallet. Nutritional value? Not much. In lieu of coffee drinks, many of the corner java spots now serve fruit cups, sandwiches, and salads with calorie counts on the packaging, which will give you the energy you need.

Skip it – do you skip lunch altogether? By blowing off lunch, your blood sugar can drop, and you won't function as efficiently. It is always smarter to eat something. Take ten minutes, and go pick up something to eat. You will be much more productive in the afternoon if you do. Studies have proven that skipping meals during the day and then overeating at the evening meal results in harmful metabolic changes in the body. As an example of the benefit of regular meals, dietitian Molly Gee, RD, MEd, (Baylor College of Medicine in Houston), cites results from studies of data from the National Weight Control Registry that showed people who successfully lost up to 72 pounds and then maintained their weight loss for five years or more were more likely to eat breakfast and to maintain a consistent eating pattern across weekdays and weekends than those who did not maintain their weight loss.

THE BROWN BAG GOES CORPORATE

Remember when you took your lunch to school? *Brown bagging it* is still in vogue today, only now there are many more benefits associated with this age-old tradition. By *brown bagging it* to work, you can control what and how much you eat so you don't gain weight.

WHAT TO DO:

Make Dagwood proud! – go for healthy sandwiches.

- Choose whole wheat bread, and make sure each slice has at least 2-3 grams of fiber. Or choose a high fiber wrap, some have up to 13 grams of fiber.
- Select flavorful lunch meats, but buy the low-sodium versions sliced for you at the deli. Turkey breast and extra lean ham have fewer calories than most other options.
- Feel like splurging? Buy some smoked salmon or make a lean steak sandwich from last night's leftovers.
- Bulk up your sandwich by stacking it with lettuce, tomato, onion, cucumber, sprouts, or whatever veggies you enjoy.
- For a total vegetarian option, make a veggie sandwich. Raw vegetables work well, but take it up a notch by grilling or roasting the veggies to enhance the flavor. Using dense vegetables such as a portabella mushroom or an eggplant in your sandwich is both nutritious and filling.
- Shake up the whole sandwich concept, and use a tortilla instead of bread to make a wrap. Place the tortilla in the microwave for 10 seconds so that it will be easier to roll – and digest. Look for the low-calorie/high-fiber types at the store.

Super soups & salads

- Soup can be a meal in itself, or a first course at lunch. You can buy soups in ready-to-microwave containers (check the label to ensure you buy the low-sodium variety). Stay away from creamy soups, and choose the broth-based types instead. If you make your own soup, bring it to work in a thermos or another air-tight container and, to avoid spillage, place your container in a baggie. *Better safe than stained!*

- Bag the salad! The best way to bring a salad to work is in a bag-gie. You can keep a plate and a metal fork at your desk (there is nothing worse than eating a salad with a plastic fork!) Keep it crisp, and pack the dressing in a separate container so you don't end up with a limp and soggy salad. Choose low-calorie, low-fat salad dressings, and watch your portions. To use less dressing, measure out 1 to 2 Tbsp, pour it in your salad bag, and shake.

Pack snacks!

Control your portion sizes by counting out healthy items and plac-ing them in plastic bags.

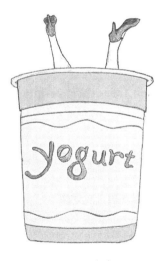

- Go for snacks like pretzels, cut vegeta-bles, and fruit.
- Fruit can double as a snack or dessert and offers great fiber.
- If you insist on a sweet dessert, be sure to limit the portion – you only need a small amount to satisfy a craving.
- To satisfy a chocolate craving, buy high-quality chocolate you can enjoy in small portions. All you need is one or two small squares. Break them in half, and place one piece in your mouth, do not bite or chew, just let it melt so you can savor the flavor. For the most flavorful chocolate check the label and buy the one with less than 12 grams of sugar.
- Bring hard boiled egg whites, raw nuts and slices of turkey for protein snacks.

WHAT TO DO LESS OFTEN:

- **Careful with the condiments** – think twice before using any condiments. Read labels to assess fat and sodium content, and avoid mayonnaise, oils, and butter, which all have about 120 calories per Tbsp. Instead, use the more diet-friendly choices, such as mustards, relishes, or salsas.

- **Geez cheese** – be careful when adding cheese to your sandwich. Most cheeses are 100 calories per slice, unless you use a low-fat version: plus you can barely taste the cheese on a sandwich anyway.

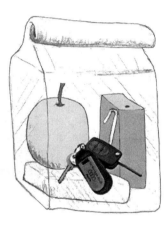

Your final challenge – now that you are packed up and ready to eat healthy for the day, your only remaining challenge is remembering to take your food with you in the morning. To ensure you don't forget, place your car keys in the bag!

Forgot to Bring Your Lunch?

Couldn't get away? Deadlines and piles of paper to conquer? Here are some great foods to keep at your desk for times when you can't leave the office or you forget to bring your lunch.

- Soups in microwaveable containers
- Boxes of raisins
- Peanut butter
- Graham crackers
- Diet hot chocolate packets that only require hot water
- Tea bags
- Almonds (10 = 100 calories)
- Tuna in pouches or cans (can be smelly so beware!)
- Rice cakes
- Low-fat 100-calorie packs
- Microwave popcorn in 100-calorie packs

The foods you keep at work for emergencies should be non-perishable and tightly sealed. You don't want to start an ant colony under your desk!

The 3 o'Clock Slump

Candy or caffeine? – not your best choice. Whether you are traveling or just having a normal day, I constantly hear that 3 to 4 o'clock is a tough time of day because people "hit the wall" or feel sluggish. Some folks go to the local java spot for a caffeine fix, while others opt for a candy bar with diet pop. However, you will be better off eating protein for energy.

Hunger or thirst? – don't forget that we often think we're hungry, but in reality we are only thirsty. Load up on some water or hot tea before eating something.

Toothbrush savior – sometimes when you are craving comfort foods, you are not really hungry, you just want to eat something to fill a void. A great trick is to brush your teeth. Once you have that refreshing mint flavor in your mouth, you will be less likely to snack.

Protein punch – sugar breeds more sugar, and diet soda encourages more sweets, better choices to re-energize you are:
- Greek yogurt eaten straight or garnished with honey or fruit
- A slice of deli turkey, ham or chicken wrapped around a pickle and you can enjoy the crunch.
- Hard-boiled eggs are another filling alternative. To make it the ultimate protein hit, lose the yolk and filled the egg white with one Tbsp of hummus...delish!
- One slice of low-sodium deli meat with a piece of low-cal cheese will also give you a boost.
- Cottage cheese by itself or with some fruit
- Nuts are a great way to boost your energy; almonds, walnuts and pecans are about 170 calories per ounce. They have good fat, but lots of calories, so portion out your own 100 calorie packs.

- Low sodium chicken broth is very satisfying and only 15 calories per cup.

Promise me produce - I would be remiss if I failed to mention fruits and vegetables, which are always your **best choice!** Dip them in hummus for a little bit of protein.

THE CHALLENGE OF FREE FOOD

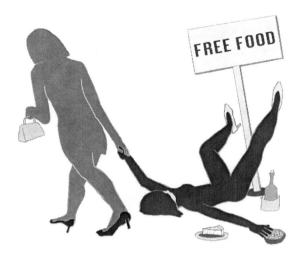

FREE FOOD – at work, there always seems to be some kind of free food for the taking. Go to a grocery store, to a big bulk store, or anywhere else, and they give out samples. Try to resist the magnetic pull these freebies generate. Unfortunately, they usually aren't worth the calories.

Office donuts – in my old office, if you won the football pool, it was your responsibility to buy donuts for the whole office. And everyone waited, like vultures, for you to arrive with the donuts in hand. Free donuts … who can say no? You can.

Recycled party leftovers – whenever someone in the office had a family gathering or party over the weekend, it was guaranteed they would arrive on Monday with a plate of wonderful treats they wanted to get out of their house. Guess what? It is not your responsibility to eat their leftovers.

Candy dishes, here, there and everywhere – and of course there are always the candy dishes people keep on their desks for everyone to enjoy. Whether there are M&M's or Good and Plenty, everyone will indulge in a handful of free candy. Best advice is not to start, because once you start, it is difficult to stop.

What is it about free food that makes us feel obligated to eat it? For some reason, whether it's due to mindless eating, hunger pangs, or any other reason, we feel a compulsion to eat free food.

GET OVER IT!

Free in dollars does not translate to free in calories!

SECTION FOUR:

ENTERTAINING, HOLIDAYS, AND SPECIAL EVENTS

Holidays and special events present excellent opportunities to spend time with those who are dear to us.

They also include our favorite foods. To eat successfully during a holiday feast, focus on the people and not on the food. Enter the holiday with a plan for what you will give yourself permission to eat and how much.

Just because it is a holiday;
It's not a license to eat endlessly.

Start your day with a plan – sound familiar?
- Eat all your meals, but keep them small so you can enjoy yourself at your special event.
- Eating smaller portions throughout the week will enable you to allow for extra calories on your special day when you aren't sure how all the foods were made.
- Wear clothing that fits snuggly so you don't feel like eating as much. If you wear a pair of sweats or any pants with an elasticized waist, that will increase your temptation to eat more.
- Eat slowly to give your stomach time to tell your brain that you are full. Chew each bite thoroughly before swallowing, and put your fork down between bites.

Bountiful buffets – if you are at an event where they are serving buffet style, first examine the real estate and see what you really want to eat. Make smart choices and *only plate your food once*. Try to limit your choices to four foods. If you use a smaller plate, it will help you to control your portions.

Establish an order – start with a salad, then eat your side veggies, then move on to your starch and protein dishes. Whether the host is serving meat, fish, or chicken, limit your portion size to 3 to 4 oz. – the palm of your hand is the best measuring tool. Remember that half your plate should be vegetables. And the more colors you eat, the more nutrients you consume!

Portion control – make it a rule that you always leave 1/3 to 1/2 of what you are served, depending on the size of the portion.

Be kind to yourself – give yourself permission to have a special treat, and plan for it. Sometimes there is something that you can't resist, like Aunt Ruth's lemon squares. Instead of depriving yourself, split one with someone or eat half and discreetly throw the other half away. You only taste the first couple of bites anyway. Don't set yourself up to fail by being so strict that in the end, you say, "To heck with it," and eat everything in sight.

Hand control – water is a great tool when you are in an "uncontrolled" situation. Drink lots. Have a sip between bites of food, and keep a glass of water in your hand at all times. Say no to picking up food with your fingers (like "drive-by" hors d'oeurves). If you have to eat with a spoon or fork, you will be more aware of what and how much you are consuming.

Manage your stress levels – whether you're the host or guest, situations can arise that cause stress. Stress can be increased by a person you will be seeing or the stress of organizing a huge event. Try not to use food as your safety net. Instead, drink lots of water, go for a walk around the block, or do something physical to relieve the stress. Eating your way through the holiday will only make you hate yourself in the morning.

Buddy system – make a pact with someone who will be there. It's kind of like having an exercise buddy to get you to the gym. Ask a friend or relative to help you stick to your plan.

SPECIAL OCCASIONS AND FAMILY DINNERS

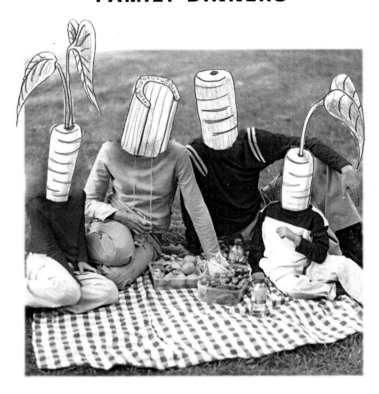

Picnics and Barbeques

Hostess gift – instead of bringing a box of candy or tray of desserts, bring a tray of cut vegetables (sold in grocery stores, ready to go) or a fruit tray. You will be able to indulge in these starters guilt-free.

When you first arrive – join in a great conversation or activity not involving food. Also remember that the longer you put off eating, the less you will be inclined to eat. Start with raw vegetables, which are crunchy, tasty, and filling.

Beverages – plan on having one or two cocktails Drink it slowly then switch to water or flavored club soda. Beer is a fan favorite at BBQs. Go lite, and save some calories. (See pages 57-59 for the "411" on drinking)

Entrées – if your host is serving hamburgers and hot dogs, you will reduce your fat and calories by choosing a turkey burger, veggie burger, or chicken breast. (You can always bring your own to throw on the grill if the host/hostess does not have alternatives). Get familiar with the numbers so you are prepared to make the best choice:
- Chicken breast without the skin (3 oz) = 142 calories
- Beef hamburger (4 oz.) = 185 calories for 95% lean meat
- Turkey burger (4 oz) = around 150 calories
- Beef hot dog = around 188 calories
- Brat = 250–300 calories
- Steak (4 oz.) = 210–280 calories (depending on fat content)

A delicious alternative for a picnic sandwich is a **portabella mushroom** in place of the burger. This delicious vegetable provides great taste and minimal calories!

Buns and condiments – it's always best to eat whole grain bread rather than white bread. Limit your calories, pitch half the bun, and eat your sandwich open-faced. Avoid mayonnaise or oil on sandwiches. Opt for mustard; there are endless options like dijon, honey mustard, and jalapeno. To add volume and flavor, add lettuce, tomatoes, sprouts, and even cucumbers. Pickles are good but high in sodium, so limit your intake.

Sides – opt for tossed salad and please control the dressing. Other favorites are grilled vegetables and corn on the cob. Grilling food adds flavor without adding butter. *Did you know that eating butter coats your tongue and keeps you from enjoying the true flavor of the food?*
- Potato salad and coleslaw are popular picnic fare. When they are made with low-cal dressing you can enjoy them in small portions. But beware of these choices when made with mayonnaise.

- If baked beans are on the menu, chose the vegetarian type that are 1 cup = 236 calories; avoid the ones made with bacon and ham.

Chips ... ahoy, oy – chips are addictive and a "waist" of calories! If chips are a must, take 5 to 10 chips and put them on a plate instead of grabbing them from the bowl and eating mindlessly. Sidestep the dips, but if you can't resist, place one Tbsp of fat-free dressing or salsa on your plate to control your calories.

Drink lots of water – you will feel full and will be less likely to overeat. Plus, it will keep you cool on a hot summer's day!

HALLOWEEN

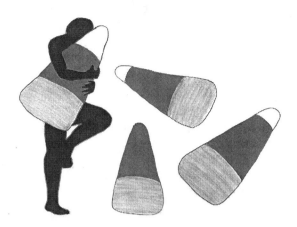

Candy is *EVERYWHERE* during the month of October and beyond—At the office, at every store and in your homes! *EEEEEEEEK!* We are talking mega-calories. How can one survive being pelted with candy from every direction? What are the alternatives? Here are some ways to "survive" this very scary holiday:

Abstinence. It's the BEST way to solve the problem, but probably not the most realistic.

Dress-up. Focus on being with friends, the costumes, and the good times associated with Halloween.

Real food first. Make sure you and your children eat dinner before ringing doorbells for too-sweet treats.

The loot. When your children come home with bags overflowing with candy, let them chose their 10 favorites; donate the rest to kids who were not as fortunate. Then spread out the sugar intake: Pack your child's favorites in their lunch each day for the next two weeks!

Candy lovers. Identify which candy you love the most and read the label. This in itself could cure your candy cravings. Eat sugar-free alternatives that satisfy you; set a limit and stay within your daily calories.

Candy corn. It can still be enjoyed if you're counting calories. Just limit your serving size to 18 pieces or less. Some candy companies make this easy with Halloween treat packs; individually packaged servings containing 6-12 pieces of candy corn are each (32-65 calories per pack). The only downside is you have to buy the 3 lb bag of treat packs - a total of 5040 calories! Use these large bags for the kids who say 'trick or treat."

Bobbing for apples. Enjoy a healthy alternative. There are 80 fiber-filled nutritious calories in each apple. Great choice!

Popcorn magic. Popcorn is a very wise and healthy choice, and provides fiber in your diet. Try spraying your popcorn with refrigerated no-calorie butter spray, then toss in some Splenda and a bit of cinnamon. Shake well and enjoy!

Toasty treat. Toasted marshmallows really hit the spot at only 20 calories each!

Party-on! Throw your own Halloween party so you can control what is served.

Oops! If you do "blow it" - no matter how badly – don't waste time beating yourself up. The most important step you can take is to get back on plan immediately. Avoid the "Oh well, I might as well wait until after the holidays" trap – there's more than enough time between now and New Year's to lose some serious weight and feel great!

Have fun! Most important, don't get so obsessed about losing weight to the point where you take the excitement out of the holiday for yourself and those around you. Use the tips from this book and develop a healthy attitude towards food. You deserve to go out and enjoy a safe, fun Halloween.

Powerful punch! Beware of holiday punch, which is usually loaded with sugar.

Ten Non-Candy Trick or Treat Items

1. Go nuts! Nuts are packed with nutrition, are safe for the teeth, and are high in calories... please control your portion.
2. Change from your change jar
3. Gift certificates for local events (bowling, arcades, pony rides, etc.)
4. Pint-sized bottles of spring water
5. Stickers
6. Erasers (be sure small children know they are not candy)
7. Pencils
8. Crayon packs and coloring sheets
9. Individual bags/boxes of sunflower seeds, pumpkin seeds, or raisins
10. Give 'em something to chew on. Sugar-free gum is still gum!

THANKSGIVING

This non-denominational holiday is so special because we celebrate what we are grateful for and enjoy the day with people we love. It is a time to focus on your friends and family versus the food. Having meaningful conversations, watching football and participating in whatever traditions you enjoy are the *true* ingredients for creating wonderful memories! However, most people equate Thanksgiving with the food. Here are some tips for surviving Thanksgiving Day:

Start the day right — exercise. Work out in the morning; get your metabolism going.

Eat first – be sure to eat something 'lite' before going to your Thanksgiving feast. When you save calories by not eating beforehand, you can sabotage yourself by getting too hungry!

Helping hands – help serve. By keeping busy, you'll have less time to nibble.

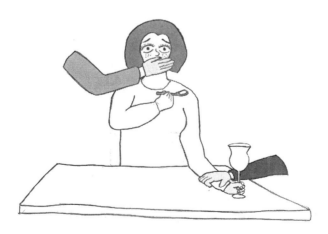

Taste testing – if you're hosting the meal, resist the urge to taste what you're making. Each taste can be 25 to 50 calories!

Cocktails? – give yourself permission to have one or two drinks. Your best choice is wine at only 20 calories per ounce. It is also okay *not* to drink alcohol!

H_2O – drink lots of water. Among the multiple benefits, drinking water makes you feel full. And when you have a glass in your hand, you won't feel left out, while others drink their calories.

Location, location, location – position yourself away from the appetizers and buffet to avoid temptation.

Beware of leftovers – make sure all of your guests go home with leftovers, especially desserts. Or you can freeze your leftovers for another time. Just make them disappear.

Walkie-talkie – ask someone to join you for a walk and chat after dinner to help your food digest. If it's cold outside, bundle up and walk fast to keep warm.

Laughter is where it's at! – most of all, have fun!

Get your groove back – over the long holiday weekend after the Thanksgiving feast, women should keep their calories around 1200. Men should keep eat no more than 1700 calories each day to compensate for the additional calories eaten.

A Reality Check: How many calories are in your Thanksgiving dinner? (I almost thought it was Halloween, I got so scared!) Get to know your number so you can make a plan.

The Star: Turkey – keep it to 4 oz. only:
- White meat, no skin (4 oz) = 178 calories
- Dark meat, no skin (4 oz) = 212 calories
- White meat, with skin = 214 calories
- Dark meat, with skin = 230 calories

Options & other sides
- 4 oz. ham = 180-240 calories
- 6 oz. candied sweet potatoes = 250 calories
- 1/4 cup gravy = 47 calories
- 1/2 cup stuffing = 178 calories
- 1/4 cup cranberry sauces = 110 calories
- 1/2 cup green beans = 17 calories
- 1/2 cup green bean casserole = 60 calories
- 1 naked medium sweet potato = 117 calories
- 1 naked medium baked potato = 161 calories
- 1 cup mashed potatoes = 237 calories
- 1/2 cup acorn squash = 57 calories
- 1 cup corn = 132 calories

Traditional Desserts:
- Apple pie (1 slice = 1/8 of a 9" pie) = 410 calories
- Pumpkin pie (1 slice = 1/8 of a 9" pie) = 316 calories
- Pecan pie (1 slice = 1/8 of a 9" pie) = 503 calories
- 1/2 cup vanilla ice cream (depending on the brand) = 150 – 340 calories
- 1/2 cup vanilla frozen yogurt = 120 calories
- 1 cup fruit = 80 calories
- 2 Tbsp whipped cream = 52 calories
- 2 Tbsp fat-free whipped cream = 5 calories

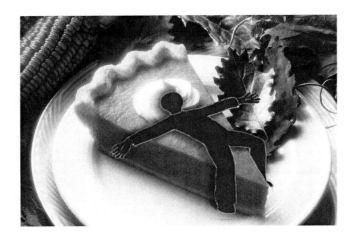

Let's celebrate!

"People are so worried about what they eat between Christmas and the New Year, but they really should be worried about what they eat between the New Year and Christmas." ~Author Unknown

Once upon a time....

Back when I was losing my weight, I went to a lovely holiday party. My strategy was not to even start on the finger foods I love, because I didn't trust myself to stop. They served rumaki, which I adore, so I decided to wait till I was leaving and take one on my way out.

Great plan!

Just as I was ready to walk over to the hors d'oeurves table, a friend says to me, "I see you eyeing that little guy!" I was shocked that he noticed and too embarrassed to take it, so I went home without my treat. Bummer. After all those years, I still crave rumaki to this day, but I hold off because it isn't worth the calories.

HOLIDAY PARTIES

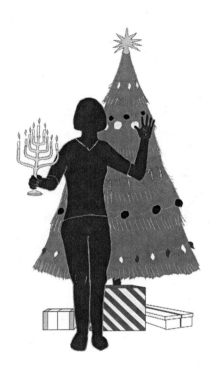

Every December we build memories and have great times. Food does not need to be the focus of your attention. Keep a diary during the holidays so you are 100% aware of what and how much you are eating. Studies have shown that you will eat less when you write down what you eat.

Balance your week – identify how many calories you should eat for the week, and then eat less on non-party days so you can indulge in some of your holiday favorites. For example, consume 1200 calories on non-event days, then eat an extra 500 calories at the party to maintain and not gain weight.

Be prepared – before any holiday party, you should eat something. Going to a party hungry is a prescription for disaster. A bottle of water and an apple are great for taking the edge off.

Finger food fooey! – each bite-sized, fat-filled hors d'oeuvre is 50 to 100 calories. They are so easy to eat mindlessly. It's better to say no, versus juggling a cocktail, a plate, a napkin and a "drive-by" hors d'oeurve. If hors d'oeurves are your guilty pleasure, stick to the veggies or the protein bites like satay (with minimal, if any, sauce) or shrimp cocktail, which are always a great choices! Make a rule not to eat with your fingers, and the appetizers are no longer a challenge.

Buffet, oy vey! – if the party has a buffet, peruse the inventory before starting a plate. Identify how you want to spend your calories, then take a plate and only fill it only once. For the best results, fill half your plate with vegetables and limit your selections to four items so you don't overindulge.

Eat small amounts of the foods you love – the last thing you want to do is leave the party feeling deprived. If you want to try a dessert or a high-fat appetizer, go for it. Just watch your portion size, eat it slowly, and savor the flavor.

Pace yourself – slow down. It takes a few minutes for your brain to realize your stomach is full. Savor the flavor, take small bites, and enjoy them. Place small portions on your plate, and realize this is all you are going to have. Set your fork down between bites and sip some water. Chew each bite thoroughly before you swallow. Enjoy the conversation at the table with your friends and family and, remember, it is just food. The memories of this or any event will be about the people, not the food.

It's not the minutes spent at the table that put on weight, it's the seconds – seconds are not an option if you are watching your waistline. But sometimes it isn't easy to resist your favorite holiday foods. Try these tips:
- Position yourself away from the buffet table.
- Delay eating for as long as possible because, once you start, it's hard to stop.
- Take your mind off food by engaging in conversation. It works for me!

Drink plenty of water – it is easy to drink 2 large glasses of water at each meal. The added bonus is you will eat more slowly and probably eat less. You can also use water (flat or sparkling) to curb the amount of alcohol you drink. Start off with water, and then alternate water with your cocktail of choice. (Please check out page 55-59 for more info about drinking!)

HOLIDAY FAVORITES

It's always a good idea to know how many calories are in your seasonal favorites:

Chanukah:
- Latkes (potato pancakes) = 100 calories for a 3 1/4" ´ 3 5/8" ´ 5/8" medium pancake
- Applesauce 1/2 cup = 50 calories
- Sour cream, low-fat 1 Tbsp = 20 calories; regular 1 Tbsp = 26 calories

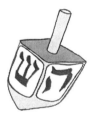

Christmas:
- Ham – 5 oz serving = 237 calories
- Turkey – 4 oz. white meat, no skin = 178 calories
- Jello mold – 1/2 cup = 100 calories
- Dinner rolls = 90-120 calories each
- Christmas cookies = 80 to 300 calories each depending on size

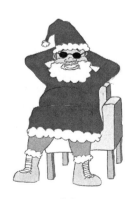

Kwanzaa:
- Fried okra – 4 oz = 238 calories
- Jamaican jerk chicken – 5 1/2 ounces = 280 calories
- Benne cakes = 54 calories per cookie
- Sweet potato pie (1 slice = 1/8 of a 9" pie) = 330 calories per slice

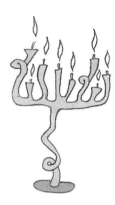

EASTER

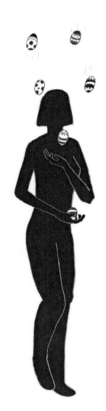

This is a time to be eggs-tremely careful about your eating. Besides the big meal, there are all those chocolate eggs and bunnies hiding out ... plus the Peeps! Because this holiday ranks a close second to Halloween for candy consumption, let's strategize on how to survive this high-fat, high-sugar holiday:

Eggs-ercise – start your day with a wonderful workout. Give it an extra 10 to 15 minutes so you can enjoy the day!

Have a plan: brunch, lunch or dinner? – your plan will determine how you manage your day. Eat a good breakfast: an egg white omelet with veggies is a great source of protein and fiber to start your metabolism. Or choose a high-fiber cereal that will keep you feeling full until the meal is served.

Be patient – whenever your gathering begins, ensure an eggs-ellent calorie-controlled day by not eating anything for as long as possible. In social situations, the longer you linger and put off eating, the better. Once you start, it's hard to stop. Start out by drinking water and chatting with relatives and friends. Check out what is being served, and only indulge in the items that are truly eggs-ceptional.. Don't eat something just because it is there.

Be egg-stremely careful all day.

- **Work the buffet** – check out what is being served, and only plate your food once. When filling your plate, set a goal of half the plate being vegetables.

- **Eat your food in order** – eat the lowest calorie foods first, and save the high-calorie foods for last. Hopefully you won't feel like eating as much by the time you get to the more fattening foods.
- **No fingers** – avoid eating foods you pick up with your fingers and eat mindlessly.
- **Seated eating only** – make it your mission to only eat when you are sitting down at the table and your food has been plated. This way you can see what and how much you are consuming, versus eating "drive-by" hors d'oeurves that can rack up 50 to 100 calories per pop!
- **Hydrate** – as always, drink lots of water throughout the day, as water makes you feel better, and it is so filling.

Now let's talk egg hunt!

Let's start with the infamous chocolate Easter eggs. These easily eaten treats are not all created equal. Read the labels (I know, I am being quite the party-pooper!), and opt for the mini-sized eggs.

Go mini – the small egg candy is one of the lightest ones around at 105 grams (3.67 ounces). While you may feel a little cheated by only indulging in a tiny egg, that mere 105 grams of chocolate heaven will still set you back 555 calories. That is equal to eating seven apples. Some of the larger chocolate eggs can be as high as 1800 calories each, and we haven't even started to talk about fat grams!

Bottom line – if chocolate is a trigger food for you, in other words, if having a taste opens the flood gates for disaster, then abstain until you are ready to leave. Then take one piece with you to enjoy on the way home. If the event is at your home, make sure all the candy leaves with your guests, and save that one piece to savor after they're gone.

Judy Weitzman

MATZO AND KNAIDLACH AND KUGEL, OH MY! (HOW TO SURVIVE THE 8 DAYS OF PASSOVER)

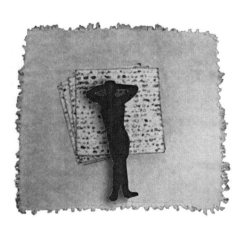

Passover is probably an extremely challenging time of the year for anyone watching their calories! It is comparable to celebrating Thanksgiving for eight days in a row! There are so many comfort foods and traditions associated with the holiday, it can make you *meshuggenah!*

WHAT TO DO:

At Passover, we make changes – since you change the dishes and the way you we eat during Passover, this would be a good time to change your exercise as well. Use the elliptical instead of the treadmill. Walk north instead of south. Take yoga instead of Pilates. Whatever you do, be sure to exercise regularly throughout this holiday.

Family-friendly time – remember to focus on your family and friends, *instead of the food!*

Cook lean – try lower-calorie versions of your favorite foods. Use egg whites instead of whole eggs, and use cooking spray instead of oil. Cut the fat in recipes.

Water works – drink lots of water and schedule lots of exercise.

Have a plan – the ritual requirements of Seder make a high-calorie night inevitable, similar to Thanksgiving. With so many courses to eat, if you just taste each, you are up to 1000 calories. For the Seder dinners, only eat what you absolutely love and enjoy. It is okay to splurge a bit at these two traditional dinners, just be careful the rest of the holiday.

Eat fresh – go with simple foods instead of all the prepared and packaged products. Indulge in seasonal fruits and vegetables, and make interesting salads. Passover is the "Festival of Spring," and both tradition and the season provide us with an opportunity for a nutritious Seder menu that includes delicious favorites and plenty of fresh fruits and vegetables.

Get lots of rest – sleep helps you stay on top of your game and, therefore, you will make smart food choices.

WHAT TO DO LESS OFTEN:

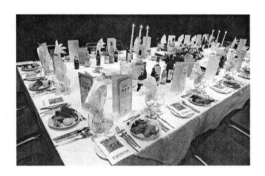

Deprivation doesn't work – don't try to totally deprive yourself of the traditional comfort foods of Pesach like kishke, potato kugel or chocolate matzo; just eat them in small portions. Give yourself permission to indulge a little bit, while controlling your eating.

Diet dilemma – don't beat yourself up if you don't lose weight during Pesach, just concentrate on maintaining your weight during this challenging week. Matzo can be binding, and there are many temptations during this unleaven week. One board of matzo is 111 calories.

Some specialty foods we eat during Pesach are foods that we should definitely eat less of, like:

- macaroons
- whipped butter
- special chocolates
- cooking with schmaltz - no longer commonplace, but still should be avoided

Recipes remodeled – many of the traditional high-calorie dishes we have enjoyed over the years can be modified to have fewer calories and less fat.

BIRTHDAYS

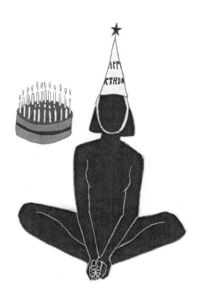

We only have one birthday per year, and it should be celebrated. There are lots of ways to celebrate a birthday without using food as the focal point.

Celebrate your day – plan a spa day, go to theatre, go for a hike, go shopping, buy yourself something new, go to a sporting event, watch a movie ... the list goes on and on.

Restaurant in your plan? – review your options. Check out the tips on page 9 on how to eat out at a restaurant.

Indulge yourself – when you are mindful of what you eat, splurging is not binging. Pre-plan how you want to spend your calories, and give yourself permission to enjoy the evening. Whether you have a chocolate martini or a piece of birthday cake or a little of both, just don't overdo it. It is no fun having a food or drink hangover.

Have a cocktail or two – no one wants to be hung-over the next day. Find more info on how to order cocktails on pages 57-59.

Eat petite – eat only until you are full. Don't let yourself overeat and end up with that stuffed feeling that makes you feel like you just want to roll home.

Share and share alike – sharing a piece of birthday cake is a great plan. Usually when it comes to sharing a dessert, two bites should be your limit. But on your birthday, give yourself permission to have a few extra tastes.

Take back control – if you do overindulge while celebrating your life, it's okay. Get back on track the next day, and you are no worse for wear. If you are like me, you like to stretch your birthday celebration over a few weeks. In that case, only give yourself permission to splurge on the day of your birthday.

SPORTING EVENTS

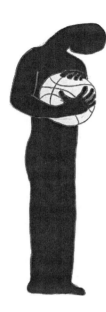

There are so many traditional treats at any sports venue that it almost seems wrong not to indulge. Here is the scoop on how to enjoy some fan favorites while cheering your team on to victory ... and still win on the scale the next day!

Beer here – the only time I even consider drinking beer is at a ballpark. The good news is the stadiums sell light beer, which is your best choice at 100 calories for a 12-oz can.

Peanuts, peanuts, who wants peanuts? – every ballpark sells peanuts in the shell. The 8-oz bag is 1280 calories and 104 fat grams!! If you can stop at 1/2 cup, you will only be consuming about 170 calories and 13 fat grams. Best plan: buy a bag of peanuts and share them with the folks sitting around you so you don't eat as many. And if no one wants any, pour some in the trash to avoid mindless eating and to control your intake.

Hot diggety-dog – the next most popular item at any sports venue is the hot dog. With the bun, we are talking around 320-450 calories, which isn't so bad.

Nachos –a fun choice, but they are deep-fried and covered with cheese. A 12 oz order is 1040 calories and 55 grams of fat....and more sodium than the FDA suggest you have for one day. Hopefully your friends will share theirs with you... a little bit will do.

Pizza by the slice – since the slices are rather large and loaded with toppings, they usually range from 500 to 900 calories per slice.

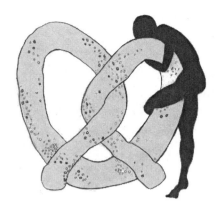

Go twist – another option is the soft pretzel, at about 450 calories it is a wonderful treat to share. Plus, it tastes great when you dip it in mustard which is calorie free.

Blue tongue or pink… not good – one bag of cotton candy rings in at 360 calories.

Expanding waistlines – the menus at most sports venues have grown over the years. You can find soft serve ice cream cones (about 230 calories per cone); Cracker Jacks (120 calories per 1/2 cup and a bag = 420 calories); and chocolate frostys in a cup (about 300 to 400 calories).

Water power! – great time to have a bottle of water or diet pop.. At Wrigley Field in Chicago, they sell bottles of water outside the park for a dollar! *Go for it!*

Bottom line: Have a plan before you go to the game; as long as it fits your day, you can eat whatever you want in small portions, And make sure you have tons of fun cheering your team onto victory!

Life Will Always Get in the Way

Excuses, excuses, excuses! – there is always going to be a birthday, special event, or dinner to attend. We can always find a reason to eat that cookie or enjoy some chips and dip. But as much as our head will give us permission to splurge, our waistlines are not as forgiving.

Spiraling out – it is only human to overeat on occasion. We can get caught up in the moment and lose sight of our goals. The trick is not letting a one-day misstep turn into a week of binging.

Here are some tips on how to regain control of your eating, before your eating goes out of control:

- Start the next day with a good workout
- Drink lots of water
- Have a good eating plan in place and stick to it
- Create a vision of yourself at your best weight to keep your goals at arm's reach
- If all else fails, try on some clothes you want to wear - the way they fit will encourage you to eat well.

The tips in this book will help you change your behaviors to ensure a healthier lifestyle. Wishing you all the best!

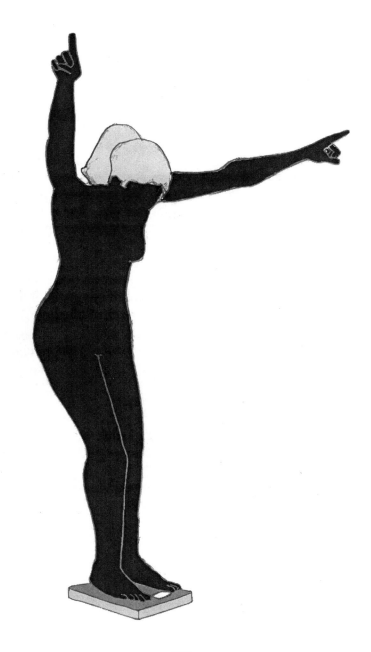